Kathryn Mannix

With the End in Mind

Dying, Death and Wisdom in an Age of Denial

WILLIAM
COLLINS

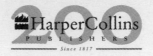

William Collins
An imprint of HarperCollins*Publishers*
1 London Bridge Street
London SE1 9GF
WilliamCollinsBooks.com

First published in Great Britain by William Collins in 2017

3

Copyright © Kathryn Mannix 2017

A catalogue record for this book is available from the British Library

HB ISBN 978-0-00-821088-5
TPB ISBN 978-0-00-824559-7

Set in Adobe Garamond Pro 11/15 pt by
Palimpsest Book Production Limited, Falkirk, Stirlinghsire

Printed and bound by CPI Group (UK) Ltd, Croydon, CR0 4YY

MIX
Paper from
responsible sources
FSC **FSC™ C007454**
www.fsc.org

This book is produced from independently certified FSC™ paper
to ensure responsible forest management.

For more information visit: www.harpercollins.co.uk/green

In a life of stories, this book is dedicated with love to the tellers of tales:

to my parents, who gave me the words;
to my husband, who distils words into wisdom;
and to our children, whose stories are still unfolding.

Contents

Introduction

It may seem odd that, after half a lifetime of keeping company with the dying, anyone should wish to spend even more time immersed in telling their stories. It may even seem presumptuous to offer those stories in the hope that readers will choose to accompany dying strangers across the pages. And yet that is what this book sets out to do.

Throughout my career in medicine, it has been clear to me that we bring our own ideas and expectations with us in any encounter with the Big Questions. Whether that is birth, death, love, loss or transformation, everyone frames their experience through the lens of what they already know. The trouble is, whereas birth, love and even bereavement are widely discussed, death itself has become increasingly taboo. Not knowing what to expect, people take their cues instead from vicarious experience: television, films, novels, social media and the news. These sensationalised yet simultaneously trivialised versions of dying and death have replaced what was once everyone's common experience of observing the dying of people around them, of seeing death often enough to recognise its patterns, to become familiar with life lived well within the limits of decreasing vigour, and even to develop a familiarity with the sequences of the deathbed.

That rich wisdom was lost in the second half of the twentieth century. Better healthcare, new treatments like antibiotics, kidney dialysis and early chemotherapy, better nutrition, immunisation programmes and other developments radically changed people's experiences of illness and offered hope of cure, or at least post-ponement of dying, that was previously impossible. This triggered a behaviour change that saw the sickest people being rushed into hospital for treatment instead of waiting at home to die. Life expectancies increased; many lives were enhanced and lengthened.

Yet these welcome healthcare advances can only remediate us up to a point; beyond the point of saving us to live 'well enough' there is a point of futility. Here, technology is deployed in a new deathbed ritual that is a triumph of denial over experience. The death rate remains 100 per cent, and the pattern of the final days, and the way we actually die, are unchanged. What is different is that we have lost the familiarity we once had with that process, and we have lost the vocabulary and etiquette that served us so well in past times, when death was acknowledged to be inevitable. Instead of dying in a dear and familiar room with people we love around us, we now die in ambulances and emergency rooms and intensive care units, our loved ones separated from us by the machinery of life preservation.

This is a book about real events. Everything described really happened to someone, sometime, in the last forty years. To preserve the anonymity of the people described, almost all the names have been changed, along with their jobs, and sometimes their gender or ethnicity. Because these are stories rather than case histories, sometimes the experience of several people is woven into a single individual's narrative, to allow specific aspects of the journey to be depicted. Many of the situations may seem familiar because, despite our averted gaze, death is unavoidable, and these accounts will have parallels in many people's own experience.

Because most of my career has been spent working in palliative care, it is inevitable that most of these stories are about people who have had access to palliative care specialists. This generally means that any challenging physical symptoms have been engaged

with and usually reasonably well controlled, and emotional symptoms are being addressed. Palliative care is not solely concerned
with dying: excellent symptom management should be accessible
to people of all diagnoses at any stage of their illness, when they
require it. That is the broad remit of the specialty of palliative
medicine. The majority of our patients, however, are in the last
months of their lives, and this gives us a particular insight into
the way people live when they know that they are dying. It is that
part of our experience that I am seeking to convey in these stories:
how the dying, like the rest of us, are mainly getting on with
living.

In the main, I am offering the reader my eyes and ears, my
seat at the bedside, my place in the conversations, and my perspective on events. Where there are lessons for us, these are the gifts
of the people whose stories are collected here. Where there are
mistakes, they are entirely my own.

It's time to talk about dying. This is my way of promoting the
conversation.

Reading the Label

Medicines usually have a label that says 'Take as directed.' This helps us to get the intended benefit from the prescription and to avoid under- or over-dosing. The prescriber should have described what the medicine is for, and agreed a dosing schedule with the patient, who can then choose whether or not to follow the medical advice. The label also often includes a health warning, to ensure that patients know about any potential hazards.

Perhaps it will help you to decide how best to approach this book if I describe what it's for, and what kind of 'dosing schedule' I had in mind. And yes, there is a health warning, too.

This book is a series of stories based on real events, and the intention is to allow the reader to 'experience' what happens when people are approaching the ends of their lives: how they cope; how they live; what matters most; how dying evolves; what a deathbed is like; how families react. It's a tiny glimpse into a phenomenon that is happening somewhere around us every single day. By encountering death many thousands of times, I have come to a view that there is usually little to fear and much to prepare for. Sadly, I regularly meet patients and families who believe the opposite: that death is dreadful, and talking about it or preparing for it will be unbearably sad or frightening.

The purpose of this book is to enable people to become familiar with the process of dying. To achieve this, the stories have been grouped into themes, beginning with stories that describe the unfolding and evolution of dying and the variety of ways in which people respond to it.

Throughout the book, each story can stand alone to satisfy readers who like to dip in and out at random, but there is a gradual progression from more concrete principles like physical changes, patterns of behaviour or dealing with symptoms, towards more abstract concepts like making sense of human impermanence and how we evaluate, in the end, what has been truly important to us.

Also threaded through the book, but not in any chronological order, is an account of my transition from a naïve and frightened student to an experienced and (relatively) calm physician. My life has been immeasurably enriched by working within clinical teams of skilled colleagues, many of whom feature in these stories. They have supported me and acted as mentors, role models and guides throughout my career, and I am deeply aware that our strength lies in teamwork, which always makes us stronger than the sum of our individual parts.

Health warning: these stories will probably make you think not just about the people in them, but about yourself, your life, your loved ones and your losses. You are likely to be made sad, although the aim is to give you information and food for thought.

At the end of each section there are suggestions of things to think about and, if you can, to talk about with someone you trust. I've based these suggestions on current knowledge from clinical research, on ways I have seen people and families coping with serious illness and death, and on the gaps I have encountered that could have been filled to make the last part of life, and the good-byes, so much less challenging.

I'm sorry if you're made sad, but I hope that you will also feel comforted and inspired. I hope you will be less afraid, and more inclined to plan for and discuss dying. I wrote this book because I hope we can all live better, as well as die better, by keeping the end in mind.

Patterns

Medicine is full of pattern-recognition: the pattern of symptoms that separates tonsillitis from other sore throats, or asthma from other causes of breathlessness; the pattern of behaviour that separates the anxious 'worried well' from the stoical yet sick person; the pattern of skin rashes that can indicate urgency and thereby save a life.

There are also patterns in the way a condition evolves. Perhaps the most familiar these days is pregnancy and birth. We know the nine-month pattern of pregnancy: the changing symptoms as morning sickness gives way to heartburn; the early quickening and later slowing of the baby's movements as the swollen belly constricts activity towards term; the pattern and stages of a normal birth. Watching dying is like watching birth: in both, there are recognisable stages in a progression of changes towards the antici-pated outcome. Mainly, both processes can proceed safely without intervention, as any wise midwife knows. In fact, normal birth is probably more uncomfortable than normal dying, yet people have come to associate the idea of dying with pain and indignity that are rarely the case.

In preparing for a birth, pregnant women and their birth part-ners learn about the stages and progression of labour and delivery; this information helps them to be ready and calm when the events begin to take place. Similarly, discussing what to expect during dying, and understanding that the process is predictable and usually reasonably comfortable, is of comfort and support to dying people and those who love them. Sadly, wise 'midwives' to talk us through the dying process are scarce: in modern healthcare, fewer doctors and nurses have opportunity to witness normal, uncomplicated dying as their practice increasingly entangles technology with terminal care.

The stories in this section describe the patterns of approaching our dying, and how recognising those patterns enables us to ask for, and to offer, help and support.

Unpromising Beginnings

It is inevitable that a career in medicine will involve seeing death. My journey into familiarity with death began with a still-warm body, and continued with the necessity of discussing the deaths of patients with their newly bereaved loved ones. It was a long way from talking about dying with people who were themselves dying, a conversation that would have been discouraged by medical wisdom when I was training, but it was an apprenticeship of sorts, and it taught me to listen. In listening, I began to understand patterns, to notice similarities, to appreciate others' views about living and dying. I found myself wondering, fascinated, and I found a sense of direction.

I first saw a dead person when I was eighteen. It was my first term at medical school. He was a man who had died of a heart attack on his way to hospital in an ambulance. The paramedics had attempted to resuscitate him, without success, and the emergency department doctor whom I was shadowing was called to certify death in the ambulance, before the crew took the body to the hospital mortuary. It was a gloomy December evening and the wet hospital forecourt shone orange in the streetlamps; the ambulance interior was startlingly bright in comparison. The dead man was in his forties, broad-chested and wide-browed, eyes closed but eyebrows raised, giving an impression of surprise. The doctor shone a light in his eyes, listened over his chest for heart or breath sounds; he examined a print-out of the ECG from the last moments that his heart was beating, then nodded to the crew. They noted the time of this examination as the declared time of death.

They disembarked. I was last out. The man was lying on his back, shirt open, ECG pads on his chest, a drip in his right arm. He looked as though he was asleep. He might just wake up at any moment, surely? *Perhaps we should shout in his ear; perhaps we should just give him a vigorous shake; he would surely rouse.* 'Come on!' the doctor called back to me. 'Plenty to do for the living. Leave him for the crew.'

I hesitated. *Perhaps he's made a mistake. If I stand here long enough, I'll see this man take a breath. He doesn't look dead. He can't be dead.*

Then the doctor noticed my hesitation. He climbed back into the ambulance. 'First time, eh? OK, use your stethoscope. Put it over his heart.' I fumbled in the pocket of my white coat (yes, we wore them then) and withdrew the shiny new tool of my trade-to-be, all the tubing tangled around the earpieces. I put the bell of the stethoscope over where the heart should be beating. I could hear the distant voice of one of the crew telling someone he would like sugar in his coffee – but no heart sounds. My observant trainer picked up the end of my stethoscope and rotated it, so that it would pick up noises from the patient and not from the world, and placed it back over the heart. Now there was utter silence. I had never heard silence so solid, nor listened with such focus. And now I noticed that this man looked a little pale. His lips were a deep purple and his tongue was visible, also dusky. *Yes, he is dead. Very newly dead. Still working out how to be dead.* 'Thank you,' I said to the pale man. We left the ambulance and walked through the orange rain back into A&E.

'You'll get used to it,' said the doctor kindly, before he picked up a new chart and carried on with his evening shift. I was perplexed by the stark simplicity, the lack of ceremony. Our next patient was a child with a sweet stuck up her nose.

There were other, less vividly remembered deaths while I was a student, but in the first month after I had qualified, I earned the hospital record for the number of death certificates issued. This was simply because I was working on a ward that had a lot of people with incurable illnesses, and not due to any personal responsibility for their deaths, please understand. I quickly became on first-name terms with the bereavement officer, a kindly woman who brought around the book of certificates to be signed by the doctor who had declared the patient dead. In just the same way as I had seen in that ambulance five years earlier, I noted the deaths of fourteen people in my first ten days (or perhaps it was the other way round); the bereavement officer quipped that perhaps I should get an award.

What the bereavement officer didn't see, though, was the massive learning curve I was climbing. Each of those certificates was about a person, and each of those people had family members who needed to be told about the death, and who wanted to know the reasons their loved one had died. In my first month of clinical practice I had twenty conversations with bereaved families. I sat with people while they wept or stared blankly into a future they could barely contemplate; I drank cups of tea-with-sympathy, brewed at Sister's instruction by one of the experienced auxiliary nurses and carried on a tray ('With a proper cloth, please!' 'Yes, Sister.') into Sister's office, which was only entered by doctors with Sister's personal permission. Bereavement visits were an exception: permission was assumed.

Sometimes I was the second fiddle, listening to a more experienced doctor talking to families about illness, death, why the drugs hadn't worked, or why an infection had torn the person away just as their leukaemia was responding. The family members nodded bleakly, sipped tea, dripped tears. Sometimes I was the only doctor available if others were in clinics, or it was after hours, and sometimes I brewed the tea-with-sympathy myself, finding the familiar routine a comfort, noticing the details of the flowery, gilded china cups and saucers that Sister provided for these most special visitors, before taking a deep breath and entering the room to give the worst news in the world.

To my surprise, I found these conversations strangely uplifting.

Families were rarely totally unprepared: this was a ward for people who had life-threatening illnesses. During these conversations I would learn so much about the deceased person, things I wished I had known while they were alive. Families told stories about their gifts and talents, their kindnesses and interests, their quirks and peculiarities. These conversations were almost always in the present tense: there was a sense of their loved one still being present in some way, perhaps while the body was still tucked in the same bed, or was being cared for somewhere else in the hospital. And then they would check themselves, correct the tense, and begin to rehearse their steps into the huge loss that was gradually, terribly, declaring itself.

Some time during my first six months I had to tell an elderly man that his wife had died. She had died suddenly, and the cardiac arrest team had been called. As is customary, her husband had been telephoned and asked to come as soon as he could, no further details given. I found him standing on the ward, outside her room, looking at the unfamiliar screen across the door and the sign saying 'Please do not enter, please see the nursing staff.' The crash team had departed, and the nurses were occupied with their drugs round. I asked if I could help, and then saw the bewilderment and fear in his eyes.

'Are you Irene's husband?' I asked. He moved his head to say yes, but no sound came out of his mouth.

'Come with me, and let me explain,' I said, leading him to Sister's office and to yet another of those conversations that change people's lives. I don't remember the detail of the conversation, but I remember becoming aware that, with the death of his wife, this man now had no remaining family. He seemed frail and lost, and I was concerned that he might need support in his bereavement. Had I been more aware then of the wonderful contribution that can be made by GPs and primary care services, I might simply have asked his permission to let his GP know that his beloved wife had just died, but I was inexperienced and in an unexpected situation: I had discovered him outside his wife's room while I was in the middle of administering the midday intravenous antibiotics for the ward. I hadn't prepared myself for a bereavement discussion.

As usual when terminating these sad conversations, I assured him that I would be happy to talk to him again if he found that he had further questions as time went by. Although I always said this, and I truly meant it, families never did come back for more information. And then I acted on impulse: I gave Irene's fragile-looking husband my name and telephone number on a piece of paper. I had never given out written contact details like this before, and his apparent indifference as he screwed the scrap of paper into a ball and pocketed it seemed to indicate that this might not be a helpful contribution.

Three months later I was working at a different hospital, now as a junior on a surgical ward, when I received a phone call from the ward sister of my previous ward, she of the tray-with-cloth and the gilded china. Did I remember that patient called Irene, she asked. She had had a call from Irene's husband, and he was most insistent that he make contact with me. She gave me a number, and I called him.

'Oh, thank you for calling me back, doctor. It's so nice to hear your voice . . .' He paused, and I waited, wondering what question might have occurred to him, hoping I would know enough to answer it.

'The thing is . . .' he paused again. 'Well, you were so kind to say I could phone you . . . and I didn't know who else I could tell . . . but, well . . . the thing is, I finally threw Irene's toothbrush out yesterday. And today it isn't in the bathroom, and I really feel she is never coming back . . .' I could hear his voice breaking with emotion, and I remembered his bewildered face, back on the ward the morning she died.

The lesson was coming home to me. Those bereavement conversations are just the beginning, the start of a process that is going to take a lifetime for people to live alongside in a new way. I wondered how many others would have called, had I given them a name and a number in writing. By now I was more aware of the network of care that is available, and I asked Irene's husband for permission to contact his GP. I told him I was honoured that he felt he could call me. I told him that I remembered Irene with such fondness, and that I could not begin to imagine his loss.

Towards the end of my first year after qualification, I found myself reflecting on the many deaths I had attended in that year: the youngest, a sixteen-year-old lad with an aggressive and rare bone-marrow cancer; the saddest, a young mum whose infertility treatments may have been responsible for her death from breast cancer just before her precious son's fifth birthday; the most musical, an elderly lady who asked the ward sister and me to sing 'Abide With Me' for her, and who breathed her last just before we ran out of verses; the longest-distance, the homeless man who was reunited with his family and transported the length of England over two days in an ambulance, to die in a hospice near his parents' home; and the one that got away – my first cardiac arrest call, a middle-aged man who was post-op and stopped breathing, but who responded to our ministrations and walked out of the hospital a well man a week later.

This is when I noticed the pattern of dealing with dying. I am fascinated by the conundrum of death: by the ineffable change from alive to no-longer-alive; by the dignity with which the seriously ill can approach their deaths; by the challenge to be honest yet kind in discussing illness and the possibility of never getting better; by the moments of common humanity at the bedsides of the dying, when I realise that it is a rare privilege to be present and to serve those who are approaching their unmaking. I was discovering that I was not afraid of death; rather, I was in awe of it, and of its impact on our lives. What would happen if we ever 'found a cure' for death? Immortality seems in many ways an uninviting option. It is the fact that every day counts us down that makes each one such a gift. There are only two days with fewer than twenty-four hours in each lifetime, sitting like bookends astride our lives: one is celebrated every year, yet it is the other that makes us see living as precious.

French Resistance

Sometimes, things that are right in front of our noses are not truly noticed until someone else calls them to our attention.

Sometimes, courage is about more than choosing a brave course of action. Rather than performing brave deeds, courage may involve living bravely, even as life ebbs. Or it may involve embarking on a conversation that feels very uncomfortable, and yet enables someone to feel accompanied in their darkness, like 'a good deed in a naughty world'.

Here's Sabine. She is nearly eighty. She has a distinguished billow of silver-white hair swept into a knotted silk scarf, and she wears a kaftan (the genuine article, from her travels in the Far East in the 1950s) instead of a dressing gown. She is in constant motion in her hospice bed, playing Patience, applying her *maquillage*, moisturising her sparrowesque hands. She drinks her tea black and derides the 'You call that coffee?' offered by the beverages trolley. She has a French accent so dense it drapes her speech like an acoustic fog. She is the most mysterious, self-contained creature we have encountered in our newly built hospice.

Sabine has lived in England since 1946, when she married a young British officer her Resistance cell had hidden from Nazi troops for eighteen months. Peter, her British hero, had parachuted into France to support the Resistance. He was a communications specialist, and had helped them to build a radio from, by the sound of it, only eggboxes and a ball of string. I suppose he may also have brought some radio components in his rucksack, but I dare not ask. Forty years later, her accent sounds as though she has just stepped off the boat at Dover, a new bride with high hopes. 'Peter was so clever,' she murmurs. 'He could do any-sing.'

Peter was very brave. This is not in doubt: Sabine has his photograph and his medals on her bedside table. He died many years ago, after an illness that he bore with characteristic courage. 'He was never afraid,' she recalls. 'He told me always to remember him. And I do, *naturellement*, I talk to him every day' – and she indicates the photograph of her handsome husband, resplendent in dress uniform and frozen in monochrome at around forty years of age. 'Our only sadness was that the Lord did not send us children,' she reflects. 'But instead we use our time for great travel and adventures. We were very 'appy.'

Her own medal for courage is pinned to her chest on a black and red ribbon. She tells the nurses that she has only taken to wearing it since she realised that she was dying. 'It is to remind me that I too can be brave.'

I am a young trainee in the new specialty of palliative medicine. My trainer is the consultant in charge of our new hospice, and Sabine loves to talk to him. From his discussions with her, it emerges that he is bilingual because his father was a Frenchman, and also a Resistance fighter. He occasionally has conversations with Sabine in French. When this happens, she sparkles and moves her hands with animation; the symmetrical Gallic shrugs between them amuse us greatly. Sabine is flirting.

And yet, Sabine is keeping a secret. She, who wears her Resistance Medal and who withstood the terror of the war, is afraid. She knows that widespread bowel cancer has reached her liver and is killing her. She maintains her self-possession when she allows the nurses to manage her colostomy bag. She is graceful when they wheel her to the bathroom and assist her to shower or bathe. But she is afraid that, one day, she may discover that she has pain beyond her ability to endure, and that her courage will fail her. If that should happen, she believes (with a faith based on 1930s French Catholicism mixed with superstition and dread) she will lose her dignity: she will die in agony. Worse: her loss of courage at the end will prevent her forever from rejoining her beloved husband in the heaven she so devoutly believes in. 'I will not be worthy,' she sighs. 'I do not have the *courage* that I may require.'

Sabine confesses this deep-seated fear while a nurse is drying those silver tresses after a shower. The nurse and Sabine are looking at each other indirectly, via the mirror. In some way, that disso-ciation of eye contact, that joint labour at the task in hand, enabled this intimate conversation. The nurse was wise; she knew that reassurance would not help Sabine, and that listening, encouraging, allowing the full depth of her despair and fear to be expressed, was a vital gift at that moment. Once her hair was dressed, her silk scarf in place and Sabine indicated that the audience was over, the nurse asked permission to discuss those important concerns with our leader. Sabine, of course, agreed: in her eyes our leader was almost French. He would understand.

What happened next has lived with me, as if on a cinema reel, for the rest of my career. It formed my future practice; it is writing this book. It has enabled me to watch dying in a way that is informed and prepared; to be calm amidst other people's storms of fear; and to be confident that the more we understand about the way dying proceeds, the better we will manage it. I didn't see it coming, but it changed my life.

Our leader requested that the nurse to whom Sabine had confided her fear should accompany him, and added that I might find the conversation interesting. I wondered what he was going to say. I anticipated that he would explain about pain management options, to help Sabine be less worried about her pain getting out of control. I wondered why he wanted me to come along, as I felt I was already quite adept at pain management conversations. Ah, the confidence of the inexperienced . . .

Sabine was delighted to see him. He greeted her in French, and asked her permission to sit down. She sparkled and patted the bed, indicating where he should sit. The nurse sat in the bedside chair; I grabbed a low stool and squatted down on it, in a position from which I could see Sabine's face. There were French pleasantries, and then our leader came to the point. 'Your nurse told me that you have some worries. I am so glad you told her. Would you like to discuss this with me?'

Sabine agreed. Our leader asked whether she would prefer the conversation to be in English or French. '*En Anglais. Pour les autres,*' she replied, indicating us lesser beings with benevolence. And so he began.

'You have been worrying about what dying will be like, and whether it will be painful for you?'

'Yes,' she replied. I was startled by his direct approach, but Sabine appeared unsurprised.

'And you have been worrying that your courage may fail?'

Sabine reached for his hand and grasped it. She swallowed, and croaked, '*Oui.*'

'I wonder whether it would help you if I describe what dying will be like,' he said, looking straight into her eyes. 'And I wonder whether you have ever seen anyone die from the illness that you have?'

If he describes what? I heard myself shriek in my head.

Sabine, focused and thoughtful, reminisced that during the war a young woman had died of gunshot wounds in her family's farmhouse. They had given her drugs that relieved her pain. Soon after, she stopped breathing. Years later, Sabine's beloved husband had died after a heart attack. He collapsed at home and survived to reach hospital. He died the following day, fully aware that death was approaching.

'The priest came. Peter said all the prayers with him. He never looked afraid. He told me goodbye was the wrong word, that this was *au revoir*. Until we see each other again . . .' Her eyes were brimming, and she blinked her tears onto her cheeks, ignoring them as they ran into her wrinkles.

'So let's talk about your illness,' said our leader. 'First of all, let's talk about pain. Has this been a very painful illness so far?'

She shakes her head. He takes up her medication chart, and points out to her that she is taking no regular painkillers, only occasional doses of a drug for colicky pain in her abdomen.

'If it hasn't been painful so far, I don't expect it to suddenly change character and become painful in the future. But if it does, you can be sure we will help you to keep any pain bearable. Can you trust us to do that?'

'Yes. I trust you.'

He continues, 'It's a funny thing that, in many different illnesses that cause people to become weaker, their experience towards the end of life is very similar. I have seen this many times. Shall I tell you what we see? If you want me to stop at any point, you just tell me and I will stop.'

She nods, holding his gaze.

'Well, the first thing we notice is that people are more tired. Their illness saps their energy. I think you are already noticing that?'

Another nod. She takes his hand again.

'As time goes by, people become more tired, more weary. They need to sleep more, to boost their energy levels. Have you noticed that if you have a sleep during the day, you feel less weary for a while when you wake up?'

Her posture is changing. She is sitting up straighter. Her eyes are locked on his face. She nods.

'Well, that tells us that you are following the usual pattern. What we expect to happen from now on is that you will just be progressively more tired, and you will need longer sleeps, and spend less time awake.'

Job done, I think. *She can expect to be sleepy. Let's go . . .* But our leader continues talking.

'As time goes by,' he says, 'we find that people begin to spend more time sleeping, and some of that time they are even more

deeply asleep, they slip into a coma. I mean that they are unconscious. Do you understand? Shall I say it in French?'

'*Non*, I understand. Unconscious, coma, *oui*.' She shakes his
hand in hers to affirm her understanding.

'So if people are too deeply unconscious to take their medications for part of the day, we will find a different way to give those
drugs, to make sure they remain in comfort. *Consoler toujours*.
Yes?'

He must be about to stop now, I think. I am surprised that he
has told her so much. But he continues, his gaze locked onto hers.

'We see people spending more time asleep, and less time awake.
Sometimes when they appear to be only asleep, they are actually
unconscious, yet when they wake up they tell us they had a good
sleep. It seems we don't notice that we become unconscious. And
so, at the very end of life, a person is simply unconscious all of
the time. And then their breathing starts to change. Sometimes
deep and slow, sometimes shallow and faster, and then, very gently,
the breathing slows down, and very gently stops. No sudden rush
of pain at the end. No feeling of fading away. No panic. Just very,
very peaceful . . .'

She is leaning towards him. She picks up his hand and draws
it to her lips, and very gently kisses it with great reverence.

'The important thing to notice is that it's not the same as falling
asleep,' he says. 'In fact, if you are well enough to feel you need
a nap, then you are well enough to wake up again afterwards.
Becoming unconscious doesn't feel like falling asleep. You won't
even notice it happening.'

He stops and looks at her. She looks at him. I stare at both of
them. I think my mouth might be open, and I may even be
leaking from my eyes. There is a long silence. Her shoulders relax
and she settles against her pillows. She closes her eyes and gives
a deep, long sigh, then raises his hand, held in both of hers, shakes
it like shaking dice, and gazes at him as she says, simply, 'Thank
you.' She closes her eyes. We are, it seems, dismissed.

The nurse, our leader and I walk to the office. Our leader says to me, 'That is probably the most helpful gift we can ever give to our patients. Few have seen a death. Most imagine dying to be agonising and undignified. We can help them to know that we do not see that, and that they need not fear that their families will see something terrible. I never get used to having that conversation, even though it always ends by a patient knowing more yet being less afraid.'

Then, kindly overlooking my crumpled tissue, he suggests, 'Shall we have a cup of tea?'

I escape to brew the tea and wipe my tears. I begin to reflect on what I have just seen and heard. I know that he has just described, with enormous skill, exactly what we see as people die, yet I had never considered the pattern before. I am amazed that it is possible to share this amount of information with a patient. I review all my ill-conceived beliefs about what people can bear: beliefs that had just scrolled through my startled and increasingly incredulous consciousness throughout that conversation; beliefs that would have prevented me from having the courage to tell Sabine the whole truth. I feel suddenly excited. *Is it really within my gift to offer that peace of mind to people at the ends of their lives?*

This book is about my learning to observe the details of that very pattern our leader explained to Sabine all those years ago. In the next thirty years of clinical practice, I found it to be true and accurate. I have used it, now adapted to my own words and phrases, to comfort many hundreds, perhaps even thousands, of patients in the same way that it brought such comfort to Sabine. And now I am writing it down, telling the stories that illustrate that journey of shrinking horizons and final moments, in the hope that the knowledge that was common to all when death took place at home can again be a guide and comfort to people contemplating death. Because in the end, this story is about all of us.

Tiny Dancer

The pattern of decline towards death varies in its trajectory, yet for an individual it follows a relatively even flow, and energy declines initially only year to year, later month to month, and eventually week by week. Towards the very end of life energy levels are less day by day, and this is usually a signal that time is very short. Time to gather. Time to say any important things not yet said.

But sometimes there is an unexpected last rise before the final fall, a kind of swansong. Often this is unexplained, but occasionally there is a clear cause, and sometimes the energy rush is a mixed blessing.

Holly has been dead for thirty years. Yet this morning she is steadily dragging herself out of the recesses of my memory and onto my page. She woke me early; or perhaps it was waking on this misty autumn morning that brought her last day to mind. She twisted and twirled her way into the focus of my consciousness: initially just images like an old silent-movie reel showing disjointed snatches of her pale smile, her pinched nose, her fluttering hand movements. And then her laugh arrived, with the crows outside my window: her barking, rasping laugh, honed by the bitter winds along the industry-riven river, by teenage smoking and premature lung disease. Finally, she drew me from my warm bed and sat me down to tell her story, while mist was still bathing the gardens beneath an autumn dawn.

Thirty years ago, arriving at my first hospice job with several years' experience of a variety of medical specialties, some training in cancer medicine and a freshly minted postgraduate qualification, I probably saw myself as quite a catch. I know that I was buoyed

up by the discovery that palliative care fitted all my hopes for a
medical career: a mixture of teamwork with clinical detective work
to find the origins of patients' symptoms in order to offer the best
possible palliation; of attention to the psychological needs and
resilience of patients and their families; honesty and truth in the
face of advancing disease; and recognition that each patient is a
unique, whole person who is the key member of the team looking
after them. Working with, rather than doing to: a complete para-
digm shift. I had found my tribe.

The leader of this new hospice had been on call for the service
without a break until my arrival in early August. Despite this he
exuded enthusiasm and warmth, and was gently patient with my
questions, my lack of palliative care experience, my youthful self-
assurance. It was a wonder to see patients I already knew from
the cancer centre, looking so much better than when they had
recently been in my care there, now with pain well controlled but
brains in full working order. I may have thought highly of myself,
but I recognised that these people were far better served by the
hospice than they had been by the mainstream cancer services.
Perhaps my previous experiences were only a foundation for new
knowledge; perhaps I was here not to perform, but to learn.
Humility comes slowly to the young.

After my first month of daily rounds to review patients, adjusting
their medication to optimise symptom control but minimise
side-effects, watching the leader discuss mood and anxieties as well
as sleep and bowel habit, attending team meetings that reviewed
each patient's physical, emotional, social and spiritual wellbeing,
the leader decided that I was ready to do my own first weekend
on call. He would be back-up, and would come in to the hospice
each morning to answer any queries and review any particularly
tricky challenges, but I would take the calls from the hospice
nurses, from GPs and hospital wards, and try to address the
problems that arose. I was thrilled.

Holly's GP rang early on the Saturday afternoon. Holly was

known to the city's community palliative care nurses, whose office was in the hospice, so he hoped that I might know about her. She was in her late thirties, the mother of two teenagers, and she had advanced cancer of the cervix, now filling her pelvis and pressing on her bladder, bowels and nerves. The specialist nurses had helped the GP to manage her pain, and Holly was now able to get out of bed and sit on the outdoor landing of her flat to smoke and chat with her neighbours. When she developed paralysing nausea in the previous week, her symptoms were improved greatly by using the right drug to calm the sickness caused as her kidneys failed, as the thin ureter tubes that convey the urine from kidneys to bladder were strangled by her mass of cancer.

Today she had a new problem: no one in her flat had slept all night, because Holly wanted to walk around and chat to everyone. Having hardly walked more than a few steps for weeks, overnight she had suddenly become animated and active, unable to settle to sleep, and she had woken her children and her own mother by playing loud music and attempting to dance to it. The neighbours had been banging on the walls. At first light her mother had called the GP. He found Holly slightly euphoric, flushed and tired, yet still dancing around the flat, hanging onto the furniture.

'She doesn't seem to be in pain,' the GP explained to me, 'and although she's over-animated, all her thought content is normal. I don't think this is psychiatric, but I have no idea what is going on. The family is exhausted. Do you have a bed?'

All our beds were full, but I was intrigued. The GP accepted my offer to visit Holly at home, so I retrieved her notes from the community team office and set off through the receding autumn mist to the area of the city where long terraces of houses run down to the coalyards, ironworks and shipbuilders that line the river's banks. In places the terraces were interrupted by brutal low-rise blocks of dark brick flats crowned with barbed-wire coils and pierced by darkened doorways hung with cold neon lights in tamper-proof covers. These palaces bore unlikely names: Magnolia

House, Bermuda Court, and my destination, Nightingale Gardens.

I parked my car at the kerbside and sat for a moment, surveying the area. Beside me rose the dark front of Nightingale Gardens. On the ground floor, a bare stone pavement ran from the kerb to the tenement block: not a tree or a blade of grass to garnish these 'gardens', which certainly never saw or heard a nightingale. Across the road, a terrace of council-owned houses grinned a toothy smile of white doors and window frames, all identical and recently painted. Some of the tiny front gardens displayed a few remnants of late-summer colour; rusting bed-frames or mangled bicycles adorned others. Several children were playing in the street, a game of catch with a tennis ball played while dodging a group of older boys who were aiming their bikes at the players. Yelps of excitement from the kids, and from a group of enthusiastic dogs in assorted sizes who were trying to join in.

I collected my bag and approached Nightingale Gardens. I needed to find number 55. An archway marked 'Odds' led to a dank, chilly concrete tunnel. My breath was visible in the gloomily lit staircase. On the landing, all the door numbers were in the thirties. Up another couple of flights I found the fifties, and halfway along the balcony corridor that overlooked the misty river, and was itself overlooked by cranes rising above the mist like origami giants, number 55. I knocked and waited. Through the window I could hear Marc Bolan telling me that I won't fool the children of the revolution.

The door was opened by a large woman in her fifties wearing a miner's donkey jacket. Behind her was a staircase leading to another floor, and beside her the living-room door swung open to reveal a diminutive, pale woman leaning on a table and moving her feet to the T. Rex beat.

'Shut the door, will you?' she trilled across to us. 'It's cold out there!'

'Are you the Macmillan nurse?' the older woman asked me. I explained that I worked with the Macmillan nurses, but that I was the doctor on call. She beckoned me inside with an arc of her chin, while simultaneously indicating with animated eyebrows that the younger woman was causing her some concern. Then she straightened up, shouted, 'I'm off to get more ciggies, Holly!' and left the flat.

Holly looked at me and explained, 'We smoked 'em all last night. Gaspin' now!' Then she invited me in, saying, 'Wanna cuppa?'

There was something childlike about Holly, with her tiny frame and her dark hair swept up into a high ponytail. Her skin shone with an alabaster clarity, stretched taut over swollen legs and a pinched face. She seemed to emanate a faintly yellow light, like a fading lightbulb. She was in constant motion, as though driven by an unseen force. Her feet danced while her hands leaned on the table; then she sat down abruptly in one of the upright chairs and began to rub her hands along her arms, along her thighs, along her calves, shuffling her bottom and nodding her head in time to the music. Alice Cooper next: Holly drummed her fingers, then played air guitar, tossing her ponytail to celebrate school being blown to pieces. Throughout, she sang along in a thin contralto embellished by occasional hiccups.

The music stopped with a click that drew my attention to the cassette player on the window ledge. These must be mix tapes she had recorded in her teens. Without the music to give shape to her movements, the choreography broke down and she simply rocked on her chair, rubbing her limbs with her thin hands and tossing her hair like an angry genie. She looked up at me, as though noticing me for the first time, and asked, 'Got a ciggie?' When I shook my head she laughed and said, 'Oops, no, you're the doctor, aren't you? You won't approooove of ciggies!' in a sing-song voice tinged with sarcasm.

'So, what's the deal, doc?' she said next. 'I feel GREAT today! I wanna sing and dance and get outta this bloody flat!' Casting her gaze around the room, she sighed heavily. 'It's like a pigsty in here. Needs a good cleaning. Amy! AMY!!!' she moved her gaze to the ceiling, brown with cigarette smoke, as though to look at Amy, who was presumably upstairs.

A teenage girl in pyjamas appeared at the living-room door.

'Mam?' she asked. 'Mam, what's all the *noise* for?' Then, catching sight of me, she whispered, 'Who's this? Where's Nan?'

'Nan's gone for ciggies. This is the doctor. This place needs cleaning. Get the Hoover over it, will you?'

Amy rolled her teenage eyes, said, 'Yeah, in a mo,' and disappeared back up the stairs just as her grandmother reappeared through the front door. Lighting two cigarettes at once, Nan held one out to Holly then stumped through to the kitchen, saying, 'I'll get the kettle on. Tea, doctor? Biscuit?'

Seated on the sofa, I watched Holly continue her interminable movements. I recognised this pattern. I just needed a bit more information.

'Holly, are you feeling restless?' I asked.

She regarded me solemnly, exhaled her smoke, and then said, 'Look, are you gonna ask a load of questions? Cos, not to be rude or anything, I've already done that with the first doctor. So it's like this – yes, I can't lie still, can't get to sleep, can't get the tunes out of my head. OK? Got the idea?'

Nan appeared with a tray of mugs filled with tea, a plate of biscuits and thickly sliced fruitcake. I have come to know such hospitality is a custom along the riverside.

'Holly's not usually so grumpy,' said Nan. 'I think she's tired. None of us got any sleep last night.'

'When would you say the restlessness started?' I asked. The women looked at each other to consider.

'It's really since you stopped being so sick,' said Nan.

Holly agreed. 'That puking was doing my head in. I couldn't keep nothing down. But now I don't feel sick I feel really kind of energetic.'

It seemed bizarre that this waif, glowing with the lemon tinge of kidney failure, her life ebbing like a fading echo, could describe herself as energetic. I asked her to hold her arms out in front of her and to close her eyes. Her arms twisted and danced before her, and she bounced her legs on the balls of her feet. When I took her hand and slowly flexed her arm at the elbow, I could feel the muscles tensing and releasing as though the joint was moved by cogwheels. Her gaze was unblinking in her doll-like face.

'When did the sickness stop?' I asked, although I already knew the answer: the day the nurses gave her a syringe-driver with anti-sickness medication for her kidney failure. The same day the restlessness began. Because the drugs that were stopping her nausea were also giving her this sense of driven restlessness: akathisia, or 'inability to sit'. She was perceiving the sense of drivenness as 'kind of energetic', and it was this that had suddenly caused her to get out of bed and want to move around.

Here's a dilemma. This young mother is close to the end of her life. Her kidney failure is so severe that many people would be unconscious at this stage, but the drug that has stopped her nausea and vomiting is also causing restlessness and a desire to get out and about. Her legs don't have the strength to hold her up, and she is in a fifth-floor flat. I don't want to stop the anti-sickness drug: her nausea would return very quickly. Yet she will exhaust her meagre energy reserves if she keeps pacing and dancing and cannot get some sleep.

There is a drug, an injection, that will reverse this restlessness and ceaseless drive to movement, without losing control of her nausea. We keep it in the hospice, and I can go back to get it. But in the meantime Holly is stir crazy, like a caged animal. How can we assuage her desire to be on the move?

'Do you have a wheelchair?' I ask. No, Holly was well enough to get up and down the stairs until two weeks ago. Then the pain kept her indoors. Then when the pain was better she was exhausted by her nausea.

'Sally downstairs has got a wheelchair,' chimes a voice from the doorway. Amy has been listening in. She is dressed now, in black tights and a neon-yellow T-shirt, stripy yellow-and-black leg-warmers and an army beret. 'We can borrow it. Where are you taking her?'

'I'm not taking her anywhere. I'm going back to the hospice to get another medicine to help with this restlessness. But while she's so restless and desperate to get out, I wondered if you'd like to take her out and around the shopping arcade down the road. Just for a change of scenery.'

Nan looks startled. Amy shouts, 'I'm going to ask Sally!' and leaves. Holly looks gratefully at me, and says, 'Well, I never expected *that*! Thanks, doc. They keep mollycoddling me, and getting out will be brilliant . . .'

After a couple of minutes, Amy taps on the window. She is on the balcony corridor with a wheelchair and two huge men in black leather jackets.

'Tony and Barry will carry her down, and we'll go round the shops!' she exclaims gleefully.

'Wait – there's no lift?' I ask, but there's no point – the seed is sown, the wheelchair borrowed, and Nan is already on the phone to Holly's sister to arrange to meet her at the shops. And I'm not about to contradict Tony and Barry, who are Sally Downstairs's sons. They are on a mission. And they are massive – only their enthusiastic smiles are wider than their huge shoulders.

I head back to the hospice, and phone the leader. I describe the scenario – the petite patient so frail, with advanced kidney failure; weaker day by day until this sudden flush of 'false energy' caused by the anti-sickness drug; my diagnosis of akathisia and my plan to treat it. After asking a few questions he seems satisfied by my examination and conclusions. He asks whether I'd like him to come with me to give the antidote and make the next plans, and although I want to be able to cope on my own, a mental picture of the smoke-stained room, the tiny dancing patient and the gigantic, leather-clad neighbours makes me glad to accept the offer. He drives to the hospice while the nurses help me to gather the drugs and equipment I will need.

The second trip to the riverside feels different. The mist has cleared away, and the afternoon is lengthening into early evening. Nightingale Gardens is in sunshine as we park outside, and there seems to be a party going on outside one of the ground-floor flats. Looking closer, I recognise Barry and Tony, the neon glow of Amy's T-shirt, and Holly in the wheelchair wearing a fluffy bright pink dressing gown and a knitted hat. Nan has her back to us in the NCB donkey jacket, and an older woman whom I take to be Sally Downstairs is sitting in an armchair on the pavement. Cans of beer are being drunk; there is laughter; people come and go from the flat. When the leader and I approach, we are waved over and greeted like family.

'Here's the lass what sent us to the shops!' shouts Holly, and shows me her newly manicured fingernails, a treat from her sister.

'Bugger of a job keeping her bloody hands still!' laughs Nan.

They have had a wonderful trip out: Holly has loved meeting and greeting friends and neighbours she has not seen for weeks, and all have admired her grit in getting out. She has bought a massive carton of cigarettes, a crate of beer and lots of crisps, and these are now being shared at the impromptu pavement party.

I explain that we need to check her syringe-driver and then give her a small dose of the antidote, to be sure it doesn't disagree with her before giving a larger dose to last overnight. We need to go up to her flat. Barry and Tony lift the wheelchair as easily as though it is a shopping bag, and carry Holly upstairs to the fifth-floor landing. Nan lets us in, and goes to put the kettle on; Holly's sister and Amy follow. I introduce the leader, and he examines Holly's arm movements to satisfy himself about the diagnosis. Tea mugs are produced for the workers, everyone else continues to drink beer. Holly knows she must stick to small volumes of fluids, so she drinks her beer from a dainty china teacup.

I wash my hands in the kitchen to prepare to give the antidote injection. Someone has tidied the flat since earlier today, and all the surfaces are gleaming. Then I insert a tiny needle under the loose skin of Holly's forearm, and give the first small dose. Conversation continues around the room; Barry and Tony depart with their mum's wheelchair; Nan and Amy settle into armchairs while Holly's sister, Poppy, sits beside me on the sofa, from where we watch Holly threading her restless way around the room, the leader beside her in case she falls. She is still describing the fun of her afternoon.

Eventually she takes a seat on the sofa beside her sister. She fidgets, but remains sitting. She gradually stops talking, and listens to the chatter around her. I can see the leader watching her intently.

'Are you sleepy, Holly?' he asks gently. She nods. Poppy and I make space for her to lie on the sofa, but she twists and turns. She is too frail to get upstairs to bed, so Amy, always the practical one, brings down the rolled-up mattress she uses when friends sleep over. Nan and Poppy make up a bed, and Holly lies down. Her eyes are closing.

'How are you feeling now, Holly?' asks the leader.

No reply. Holly snores gently, and Amy laughs, but Nan leans forward and says, 'Holly? Holly?!' She is afraid.

The leader sits on the floor beside the mattress and takes Holly's pulse. She is lying completely still now, breathing gently and occasionally snoring. The leader looks up at us all, and says, 'Can you see how she is changing?' And she is. She is becoming smaller. Her energy is gone, and the weariness that has been creeping up on her for the last couple of weeks is now over-whelming her.

Nan reaches for Holly's hand, and says, 'Amy, get your sister.'

Amy looks perplexed. Her sister is at a friend's house for the weekend. She won't want to be disturbed. Amy has not understood what is happening here.

'Amy,' I say, 'I think your mum is so very tired that she may not wake up again.'

Amy's mouth drops open. Her eyes dance between her mother, the leader taking her pulse, her Nan, and my face. 'It wasn't what she did today that tired her out,' I say. 'What you helped her to do today was fantastic. But she was already exhausted before her busy night last night, wasn't she?'

Amy's wide-eyed stare makes her look very like her mum as she nods in agreement. 'And that exhaustion is caused by her illness, not by how busy she's been today,' I explain. 'But if your sister wants to be here for her mum, then now is the time to come.'

Amy swallows and gets to her feet. She picks up a notebook and begins to look for a phone number.

'Give it to me,' says Nan. 'I'll phone.'

Amy silently points out the number, and Nan moves across to the window ledge, where the phone sits beside the cassette player. She dials. We hear the buzzing drone of the ring; we hear a voice answer the phone; then Nan gives her message as Holly opens her eyes and says, 'Why am I lying down here?'

'Too drunk to get to bed again,' says Poppy, trying to smile but with tears running down her nose.

'Don't cry, Poppy,' says Holly. 'I'm OK. I'm just so tired. But haven't we had a lovely day?' She wriggles herself into the eiderdown and says, 'Where's my girls?'

'I'm here, Mam,' says Amy, 'and Tanya's on her way.'

'Come and snuggle down with me,' smiles Holly. Amy looks up at us. The leader moves back to leave space and nods at her. Amy lies down alongside her mum, and hugs her.

The front door bangs open, and a girl shoots through it.

'Mam? Mam! Is she here? Where is she? Nan? Nan! What's happening?'

Nan walks over and hugs her, then draws her across the room, saying, 'She's here, Tanya, she's here. She's so tired we've made her a camp bed. These are the doctors. Mam's OK, but she's very tired, and she wants a cuddle.'

Tanya kneels on the floor by her mother's head, and Amy

reaches up to take her hand, drawing it down to touch their mother's cheek.

'Here's Tanny, Mam,' she says. Holly puts her hand over the girls' hands, and sighs.

Over the next half-hour, the light fades outside and the room becomes dark. No one moves. We sit in the semi-dark, an orange glow lighting the room from the streetlamps outside. Every now and then, the leader gives a quiet commentary.

'Look how peacefully she's sleeping.'

'Can you hear how her breathing has changed? It's not so deep now, is it?'

'Have you noticed that she stops breathing from time to time? That tells me that she is unconscious, very deeply relaxed . . . This is what the very end of life is like. Just very quiet and peaceful. I don't expect she will wake up again now. She is very comfortable and peaceful.'

And then Holly's breathing becomes too gentle to float a feather.

And then it stops.

The family are so mesmerised by the peace in the room that no one seems to notice.

Then Nan whispers, 'Is she still breathing?'

The girls sit up and look at Holly's face.

'I think she stopped breathing a few minutes ago,' says Poppy, 'but I was hoping it wasn't true.'

'Did you feel her move at all?' the leader asks the girls, and they shake their heads as their tears begin.

'Well done, you lovely family. You gave her the most wonderful day and the most peaceful evening. She has died' – the girls gasp and sob, and he waits for quiet before he continues. 'She has died so peacefully because she felt at peace with you here. You have done her proud.'

The girls move away from the mattress. The leader encourages them to touch their mum, to talk to her, to maintain the calm in the room. I am fascinated to see them lie down beside her again, weeping gently and whispering their love to her. It is almost unbearably sad, but this is not my family, and I feel my tears would be misplaced. I struggle to focus on the guidance being provided by the leader.

To Nan he says, 'We need to telephone an on-call GP to certify her death, and then you can call a funeral director. But there's no hurry. Give yourselves time. I'll call the doctor now. She can stay here all night if that helps you and the girls.'

Nan knows what to do. She has buried two husbands and a son.

She offers us more tea, but the leader has informed the on-call GP of the death, and says we must be going. We let ourselves out of the smoky flat and onto the lamp-lit balcony, walk in silence down the gloomy stairs and out onto the pavement.

'You OK?' asks the leader.

Of course I'm not. I think I just killed someone. 'Yes, fine,' I reply.

'You know the injection didn't kill her, don't you?'

'Mmmm . . .' I sniff.

'She was so exhausted that she would probably have died last night if she hadn't got that false energy from the akathisia. If you hadn't controlled it she would simply have danced herself to death, agitated and upset. Instead, you managed her restlessness. And that gave her the peace to lie down and cuddle her girls, after her magnificent last day.'

We walk back to the car as a new mist rolls up from the river, and evening turns to night. My first day on call for the hospice. Not a day I will ever forget.

I learned a very important lesson watching the leader talk Holly's family through the sequence of changes as her body relaxed, and dying displaced the restless energy she had been given by her anti-sickness medication. He was naming what they could observe; he was leading them through the process; he was reassuring them that all was expected, and usual, and safe. This is the task of the experienced midwife, talking the participants through the process, delivering them safely to the expected place. It is a gift that allowed the daughters to remain present and involved, and enabled them to look back and know that their calm presence was their final gift to their beloved Mam. It was a rare opportunity to watch a master at work, and to learn from that gentle, observant example.

Wrecking Ball

Watching people approaching an anticipated death offers families and friends a comfort as they all arrange their priorities and live each day as it arrives. Sometimes, though, death arrives unannounced and unanticipated. In some circumstances this is seen by the survivors as a blessing, although adjustment to sudden death is often harder than a bereavement when there has been a chance to say goodbye.

Perhaps the cruellest circumstance, though, is when a sick person has been getting better and seems to be 'out of danger', only to be snatched by death in a completely unforeseen manner. When this happens, a shocking adjustment has to be made by loved ones – and by professionals too.

Alexander and his brothers, Roland and Arthur, were named after heroes. Their mother had hoped that this would inspire them, but Alex shortened his name at school to avoid the taunting his older brothers endured daily. Alex was a quiet soul. He liked art and rock-climbing; he preferred his own company; he loved colour and texture, finding deep pleasure in creating huge canvas artworks that begged to be touched and stroked; he relished the challenge of solo climbs on solitary pinnacles. Eschewing his family's encouragement to train as an accountant, he took up an apprenticeship as a painter. He neither captured continents nor courted fair damsels: he could feel his mother's tense anxiety for his future.

But there were heroic aspects to Alex. He was tenacious and determined about his art, and he tolerated physical discomfort without complaint. He endured pain in his back for months, thinking he had pulled a muscle while moving ladders. Only when he was unable to help his boss paint a ceiling because of his pain did he consult his GP. He was then passed between health professionals for six months before someone X-rayed his chest. The X-ray showed a snowstorm of golf-ball-sized cancer masses throughout Alex's lungs. And then the penny dropped.

'Alex, before all of this back pain and tiredness started, did you ever have any pain in your scrotum, or feel a lump in one of your testes?' asked the doctor who had ordered the X-ray. Alex had not anticipated such an odd question, but he could clearly remember that several months previously he had had a 'hot, sore ball' for a few weeks. He had thought it was a football injury, and was too embarrassed to seek medical advice. He just waited for the swelling to disappear – which it did, although his testis continued to feel hard and misshapen, and he remained too shy to mention it. Then his back pain had distracted attention from it. All that time, a cancer that had begun in his testis had been slowly spreading up the chain of lymph nodes that lies deep in the abdomen and close to the spine, causing the lymph nodes to swell and hurt, and eventually allowing the cancer cells to escape into his bloodstream and invade his lungs.

Alex arrived as a new boy to the Lonely Ballroom, the six-bedded bay where our crew of young men with the same cancer, testicular teratoma, assembled for their regular five-day infusions of chemotherapy. He was anxious, of course. Like all the visitors to the Lonely Ballroom, Alex had the cancerous testis removed and a range of scans and blood tests to detect how far his cancer had spread. It had found its way into not only his lungs, but also his liver and kidneys, and tumours were scattered around the abdominal cavity like pearls from a broken string. Getting his treatment started was urgent. And now here's the good news: testicular teratoma can be completely cured, and even when it is widely spread, the cure rates are very high. In our hospital in the 1980s, that treatment took place in the room dubbed the Lonely Ballroom by its brotherhood of occupants.

Waiting for his drip to be set up on his first day, Alex paced restlessly around the ward and up and down the high, glass-walled staircase, from which there is a great view of the locality: the huge, rolling green park near the city centre, the roofs and chimneypots on the terraces of local houses, and the Victorian cemetery at the back of the hospital. The cancer centre was built with its windows facing away from the cemetery (*Don't mention the D-word*), but all our patients could see it as they parked their cars or disembarked from their ambulances and came up the staircase to the wards.

Teratoma is a cancer of young men. When Alex was shown to his bay, he found five companions already comparing notes on how their last three weeks had gone, debating whether the local football team would ever get off the bottom of the league table, and whether bald can ever be sexy – of specific importance to young men whose chemotherapy had rendered their heads as shiny as polished eggs. They all had drips in one arm and, dressed in shorts and T-shirts, were lounging on their beds or walking around with their drip stands, sharing magazines and chewing gum. They were waiting for their first dose of anti-sickness medication, after which the saline bags on their drip lines would be replaced by bags of chemotherapy. They welcomed Alex like a brother.

'Which side, mate?'

'Spread far?'

'Tough luck, mate, but they'll see you right in here.'

'You gonna shave your head or just wait for your hair to drop out?'

I was the most junior doctor in the cancer centre, and I was attached to this thirty-two-bedded ward. Drawing the curtains around Alex's bed for privacy, I explained the way the chemotherapy would be given. The other five young men in the room gathered in the far corner and continued to discuss last night's TV and the football World Cup in Mexico, in voices loud enough to demonstrate that they were not eavesdropping: each of them had, in his turn, once been here for the first time, scared and embarrassed and embarrassed to be scared; each had learned the dark humour of the cancer ward and of the Lonely Ballroom. It wasn't just the remaining testis that was lonely.

All the Lonely Ballroomers were participating in clinical trials. Data were (and still are) gathered from centres all over Europe, and it is this constant, trans-European collaborative effort to find the highest possible cure rate that has made it possible to expect cure in more than 95 per cent of teratoma patients; even people with cancer as advanced as Alex's have a cure rate of over 80 per cent. Their chemotherapy is highly toxic, not only to their cancer cells, but also to their bone marrow, kidneys and other organs.

During this arduous treatment, the hardest toxicity to bear is nausea. These boys are really, really sick: they vomit and retch and feel horribly nauseated for the full five days. Far better drugs are now available to manage treatment-induced sickness, but back then we had a cunning plan to reduce their experience of nausea: for the full five days they were given a mind-bending combination of drugs that included high doses of steroids, a sedative, and a drug related to cannabis. This made them sleepy, happy and very high. Random laughter and ribald jokes became the norm once the drugs began to disinhibit them. The Lonely Ballroom may have been a cancer ward, but it was always a cheerful one, and as the drugs wore off on day five, the guys could remember remarkably little about the experience apart from their mellow fellowship.

I explained all this to Alex, who had been told it all in clinic, but as is often the case with shocking news, he had retained only a little: *cancer, everywhere, chemotherapy, blood tests, sperm count, bald, sick, off work*. Helpful details like *curable, optimistic, getting back to work*, had simply gone over his head. He was terrified, and ashamed of being terrified; like all mountain climbers, he could face the fear of a fall and sudden death, but the idea of watching as death approached, helpless as the sacrificial virgin tied to the stake to await the dragon, was paralysing. He should be a hero like his namesake, not a helpless victim. He felt his fear and labelled himself a coward. His shame outweighed even his fear.

Laughter from beside the windows: 'Butch' Wilkins, the England midfielder, was being interviewed on TV and had just been asked whether coping with the harsh tackles sprung on him by other teams' defenders took balls. Cue belly-shaking laughter from the men with surgically adjusted tackle and single balls. Vicious humour was their weapon of choice in public. Behind the curtain, Alex regarded me with sorrowful eyes, slid down the bed while raising the sheet towards his chin, and whispered, 'I can never be as brave as them . . .' as a tear rolled slowly down his cheek.

'You only need to get through this a day at a time,' I began, but he started to rock backwards and forwards, gulping and trying desperately to remain silent as he was overtaken by sobbing. The window boys diplomatically turned the TV up. They knew, so much better than me, how the fear of the fear is the worst aspect of all.

I feel so helpless and inept. Is crying in front of me even more undermining for him? If I leave now, will that look like abandonment?

I could feel my cheeks burning, and my own eyes brimming with an overwhelming sense of helplessness before the immensity of Alex's struggle.

I mustn't cry, mustn't cry, mustn't cry . . .

'I just can't imagine how hard this is for all of you in here,' I said. 'All I know is that everyone looks like you on their first day. They all did – and look at them now.'

'I'm such a coward,' he whispered as he continued to rock, his sobs abating.

Lost for words of comfort or of hope, I reach for my tray of kit to set up Alex's drip, and he holds out both arms as if to be handcuffed.

'Are you right- or left-handed?' I ask, and like so many artists he tells me he is left-handed. While I prep the skin, tighten the tourniquet and look for a suitable vein, I ask about his art, and he tells me how much he loves the creative process: imagining the work, almost feeling it as a reality; building each canvas, layer by layer and colour by colour; how he dreams in textures and surfaces as well as pictures and colours, endlessly fascinated by the combinations of surface and space, colour and blankness that he sees in nature when he is walking and climbing. He is completely transported as he speaks, and in minutes his drip is attached and his face is calm. I ask permission to pull back the curtains, and we see his five room-mates playing cards beside the TV, a circle of shiny heads and drip stands like a peculiar toadstool ring sitting in a copse of metallic trees.

'Want to join in, mate?' one of them asks. Alex nods, and grabs his drip stand. I escape to ponder whether bravery is about being fearless or about tolerating fear. *Why do the ideas for helpful responses arise only as I walk away from the bed?*

By late afternoon, all the lads are high as clouds and vomiting for England. They lie on their beds and attempt to aim their laid-back heads towards the washing-up bowls that are provided for them: they are too sleepy and slow to catch sudden vomits in the small plastic kidney bowls used for the rest of the ward. They laugh at each other and cheer each other on, and by the time I head for home they are all singing along tunelessly to that year's World Cup song – which may not, in fact, have had a tune anyway.

Three weeks pass, and it's another Monday in the Lonely Ballroom. Six lots of blood tests to collect; six drips to set up; six sets of mind-altering drugs to prescribe; six reviews of the last three weeks. Alex is no longer a new boy; he knows the drill, and his shiny head now matches his room-mates'. There is shared outrage at Maradona's 'hand of God' goal against England. Alex's chest X-ray shows that his many cancer deposits are shrinking very quickly. I take the big, grey transparencies to show him, and he is intrigued by the images, by the contrast of dark and light, the puffball shadows looming large and white against the dark lung tissue, and the huge reduction in size after only the first round of chemotherapy. I explain that all the other secondary deposits in his liver, kidneys and abdomen will be doing the same thing: shrinking away as the chemotherapy has its effect. This increases his chances of cure even further. He nods, serious and thoughtful. I wonder about asking how he feels in himself, whether his fear is still so raw, but I am afraid I may undo his mask, and that he may not wish to go there. I move on to the same, yet always completely different, conversation with each of the other patients.

That week, I was on call on Wednesday evening. I always inspected the Lonely Ballroom drips before going home, because if any failed during the night I would have to drive back and resite them. The guys were quiet. England were on their way home from Mexico, there was a heatwave and the ward windows, facing south, turned the room into a hothouse that was only just cooling as the evening wore on. Most of the drips looked fine, but Alex's skin was becoming slightly red around the drip-site, and he noticed that when he moved his arm, the drip stopped, causing an alarm to sound. I gathered a kitbox, pulled the curtains and set about resiting the line.

'I still don't know how to bear this,' he said softly once the curtains were drawn. *The 'happy drugs' have taken his guard down.* 'I mean, I know it looks as though I'm getting better, but even if it all goes away, we don't know that it will never come back, do we?'

I was trying to thread a plastic tube into a vein in his forearm, too focused to respond. Into the silence, he sighed, 'I can't bear waiting. How do people bear it if they're waiting to die? I wouldn't want to know.'

I taped the tube in place and pressed the button to restart the drip. The 'on' light winked encouragingly. I sat back and looked at Alex. He lay against his pillows, bright-eyed with the absence of eyelashes and brows. He looked very relaxed, yet he was scowling to try to hold the threads of his thoughts.

'Do people realise when they're dying?' he asked languidly. The

effect of the drugs would mean that, however useful our conversation might prove to be, he was unlikely to remember it. Yet in
the here and now, helped by the deep relaxation induced by his
drugs, Alex was genuinely asking about the things he feared the
most. *This is a chance that might not arise again.*

I sit still and wait. A change comes over Alex's face. He pauses,
looks up at the curtain rail, and squints as though trying to focus.
Then he says, very slowly and deliberately, 'I'm not sure whether
to tell you this . . .'

Pause. *Don't interrupt. Let him keep his train of thought.*

'Have you looked out of the windows here?' he asks eventually.

Oh no, is this about the view of the cemetery?

'Yes . . .' Cautious response. *Where are we going?*

'So you know how high it is, right?' he drawls.

I do. *I climb those stairs many times a day.*

'And you know I'm a climber, yeah?'

Yes . . .

'I've been thinking. I don't need to wait. It's an easy traverse
from the window ledges to the corner of the building. If you
dropped from there, you'd hit the concrete full-on. Like, over in
a second. Bam!' His extended arm bangs the bed, and I jump.

*Oh, dear goodness: he's worked out a suicide plan to avoid waiting
to die.*

'You've been thinking about that a lot?' I ask, holding my voice
as steady as I can.

'First thing I noticed when I arrived. Then I checked the stair-
well too. But too many things to hit on the way down – too
narrow. Outside's better.'

'And when you think about that, how does it make you feel?'
I ask, dreading the reply.

'Strong again. I have a choice. I can check out – bam!' – he
whacks the bed again, but I am ready this time – 'any sweet time
I choose . . .' He lolls back on the pillows, grinning and locking
his eyes on mine to assess my response.

'And do you think you might need to do that . . . um . . . soon?' I ask, desperately wondering how I would summon help if he bounded out of bed now and tried to squeeze through the window.

'Nah,' he smiles. 'Not now we know the bugger's on the run. But if it comes back, I won't hang around for it to mess with me.'

'So should I be worried about you doing it this week?' I ask, but he is sliding back into sleep. Within minutes, he is snoring. Tomorrow I will need to ask the liaison psychiatry team for advice, but for tonight I can see that Alex is too sleepy to move from his bed. I can go home.

The bedside phone rings in the early hours. Stupid with sleep, I answer the hairbrush before identifying the phone set. I can barely say 'Hello . . .' before the voice of our night-time charge nurse interrupts me.

'Alexander Lester!' he barks – he's ex-army. 'Bleeding both ends. Have called ICU team. Just letting you know!' The phone rings off.

What? What has happened? Why is he bleeding? His blood counts were fine. He must have done something. Has he jumped? Oh, hell – what if he's jumped? Where are my shoes? Car keys? What's going on?

It is a five-minute drive to the hospital, less at 2 a.m. with no traffic. I park in an ambulance bay and run up the stairs to avoid the Lift of Unreliability. Panting and sweating, I arrive on the ward to find the charge nurse striding along the corridor.

'Ah, Dr Mannix, ma'am! Patient has been transferred to ICU as I came off the phone. Blood pressure unrecordable. Fresh red blood in vomit and per rectum. Extra IV access established and fluid resuscitation commenced. Family informed. Anything else, ma'am?'

'What happened?' I ask, bewildered. 'Did he jump? Where is he bleeding from?'

'Jump? JUMP?' barks the charge nurse, and I myself jump, as if commanded. 'Whaddayamean, jump?'

I take a deep breath and say, 'Just tell me exactly what happened,' as calmly as I can.

The nurse describes how Alex was restless around midnight, then asked for a commode, then passed a very bloody motion and dropped his blood pressure, then began to vomit what looked like fresh blood. *No jumping. If I knew he was considering it and took no action, it would be my fault.* Mixed waves of relief and alarm struggle for supremacy, and are trounced by a tsunami of guilt: *I am worrying about myself when Alex is in ICU.*

'Looks like he's having a massive GI bleed,' continues the nurse. 'Blown through to a major blood vessel if you ask me.'

That doesn't sound good. Ascertaining that I am not needed for other patients in the cancer centre, I am propelled by a mixture of concern and shame up the over-illuminated hospital corridor to ICU. They have called Alex's consultant oncologist, who is on his way in.

Alex lies on his side, unconscious; the room smells of bloody poo, a sweet, clinging aroma that I recognise and dread. He has two drips, one into a neck vein; his monitor shows a rapid pulse with a very low pressure. *This is bad.* A nurse keeps pressing the 'low pressure' alarm to silence its insistent shrieking. Pale beside the bed sits his mother; alongside her, a young man ('Roly,' he says briefly) looking very like a second Alex is shredding a polystyrene coffee cup. The ICU consultant is in the room. She is explaining that Alex has lost a huge amount of blood, that they are waiting for a cross-match from the blood bank because he must have virus-screened blood during his chemotherapy, that they are giving clotting factors and plasma, but that he is very, very sick, and not fit enough for surgery to try to stop the bleeding. *This is really bad. We are curing his cancer – how can this be happening?*

And then Alex's head is thrown back, almost as though it is a voluntary movement. A huge, dark-red python slithers rapidly out of his mouth, pushing his head backwards as it coils itself onto the pillow beside him; the python is wet and gleaming and begins to stain the pillowcase and sheets with its red essence as Alex takes one snoring breath, and then stops breathing. His mother screams as she realises that the python is Alex's blood. *Probably all of his blood.* Roly stands up, grabs her and removes her from the room, accompanied by the nurse. Her sobbing screams become more distant as she is led away to a quiet room somewhere.

I am stunned, paralysed by horror. *Is this real? Am I still asleep, dreaming?* But no. The coiled python is collapsing into itself like a large, maroon blancmange. Alex would appreciate the dense colour, the changing texture, the dark-meets-white on the bedding. *Shouldn't we do something? What?*

The ICU consultant seems to be far away, as though on a cinema screen, as she checks Alex's pulses and says, 'Not a good way to go . . .' Attempts at resuscitation would be futile. She shakes her head, then offers me coffee, which seems strangely calming, and I accept. We meet Alex's oncologist as he arrives, and sweep him up with us to the staff room for coffee and debrief. The oncologist has seen this before: beads of tumour that have glued gut to large blood vessels, shrinking to leave a hole as the cancer responds to the chemotherapy, channelling the whole blood volume out of the body. It is rare but recognised, and untreatable if the bleeding is massive.

And I keep thinking, *He didn't want to see it coming. He got his wish.*

Yet I know that, after the serpentine blood clot has been removed, the bedding changed and Alex's body washed, and his family are allowed to see him to say goodbye, they will find no comfort in the notion that he will never need to jump from a high building to escape the fear of knowing that he is dying. Alex has left the building, without ceremony or leave-taking. But the absence of farewell will be a lifetime burden for the little family of heroes.

And in the morning, we will need to tell the Lonely Ballroom occupants that Alex has finished his treatment.

This was a hard story to tell, and probably shocking to read. While most dying is manageable and gentle when it approaches in an anticipated way, the truth is that sudden and unexpected deaths do happen, and not all of them are 'tidy'. Although loss of conscious-ness during a sudden death usually protects the dying person from full awareness of the situation, those around them retain memories that may be difficult to bear.

Bereaved people, even those who have witnessed the apparently peaceful death of a loved one, often need to tell their story repeat-edly, and that is an important part of transferring the experience they endured into a memory, instead of reliving it like a parallel reality every time they think about it.

And those of us who look after very sick people sometimes need to debrief too. It keeps us well, and able to go back to the workplace to be rewounded in the line of duty.

Last Waltz

The vigil around a deathbed is a common sight in palliative care. In some families it is peaceful; in some there are rotas and care-for-the-carers as well as care for the dying; in some there is vying for position — most bereaved, most loved, most needed, most forgiven; in many there is laughter, chatter and reminiscence; others are quieter, sadder, more tearful; in some there is only a solitary sitter; occasionally it is we staff who keep the vigil, because our patient has no one else. So I had seen it many times before I had the perspective-changing experience of sitting at the bedside of someone I loved dearly, and would miss greatly, for the first time.

Well, this is unexpected.

The room is dark. A nightlight above the door casts a dim glow over the four beds and their sleeping occupants. Occasional muttered mumbles or stertorous snores from the other three beds emphasise the silence of the white-haired woman in the bed before me. I am perched on the edge of my chair, gazing at the pale face on the pillow, her eyes closed, her lips moving gently with each breath in and nostrils flaring briefly with each breath out.

I am searching her face for clues. A slight flicker of an eyebrow movement — is she wakening? Is she in pain? Is she trying to speak? But the metronome of the breath in, breath out continues unflurried. Unconscious; unaware; untroubled.

This is my grandmother. She is nearly one hundred years old. She has seen wonders in a lifetime lived in step with the twentieth century: as a girl, she watched as the lamplighter lit the gas lamps outside her home, and admired the dresses and evening capes as her neighbours boarded horse-drawn hansom cabs for a night on the town; as a teenager, she saw her brother falsify his papers to be allowed to fight in France, and welcomed home the hollow remnant of him that returned, twitchy and restless, after six months as a prisoner of war carrying German shells to their front line; as a young wife she saw the Great Depression, the death of one son from a disease now prevented by routine infant immunisation provided by the National Health Service, and later the death of her husband from an infection now treated simply by antibiotics that had yet to be invented then; she accompanied her remaining children into evacuation in the countryside during the Second World War, working in a munitions factory where the women on the production line twisted the detonator wires of occasional bombs in the hope that civilian lives in Germany would be spared; and then returned to her inner-city home through which an unexploded German incendiary bomb had dropped, its own detonator inactive thanks to unknown sisters in Germany. She saw the birth of the NHS; her children had access to higher education; she watched men walk on the moon. She is the matriarch of a family that now counts four living generations. And she is dying.

She draws a sharp breath in, and mutters on the out-breath.

'Nana? It's all right, Nana. We're taking you home tomorrow. You can sleep now. The rest of us are here.'

I listen. I mean I really, really listen. Are there words in the muttering? Is she dreaming? Is she awake? Is she afraid?

The monotonous rhythm of unconscious breathing returns. I sit and gaze, searching for clues in this dear, familiar face.

I have seen families keeping this watch, maintaining this searching vigil, many times. I have been working in palliative care now for eleven years, watching deathbeds on a daily basis. How can I have been so unaware of the deep, analytic attention of the families who sit and wait? This is not a passive activity; I am actively, keenly alert, probing her face for clues, interrogating every breath for evidence of – what? Discomfort? Contentment? Pain? Satisfaction? Serenity? This is the vigil, and suddenly I am encountering its familiar pattern of gathered family, and sitting rotas, and detailed reporting of almost no information, from an utterly new and unexpected perspective.

I happen to be in my home city to deliver a lecture. I was delighted to accept the invitation, because it would give me a chance to stay with my parents and to visit other family members. Then, while I was on my way here a few days ago, the family called from the hospital to ask me to divert my journey. Instead of sharing a meal at my parents' home, we assembled in a cubicle in the city hospital's emergency department around Nana's uncomplaining smile. Here, her back pain was assessed, her large but unsuspected colon cancer was finally identified, a bed was found in this bay, and once I had managed to convince the shiny, newly qualified ward doctor that painkillers would be appropriate, the hospital's palliative care team arrived to give their expert and welcome advice, so that I could be simply one of her grandchildren.

The next day, we palliative care professionals met again at the conference they had invited me to address. I stepped out of 'family anxiety' and into 'conference speaker' mode for two welcome hours of respite from my sadness, leaving a small posse of the family with Nana. The speaker after me was a social worker whose moving talk about bereaved families pierced my armour; I paused in the ladies' cloakroom to remove the mascara stains from my cheeks, and rushed back to the hospital. The posse reports that Nana has had 'tests'. She has widespread cancer. She wants to return to her nursing home, because it has a chapel and being close to God is her top priority. She is not alarmed – she has been preparing to die for decades, and has astonished herself with her own longevity, the solitary survivor of her generation and lonely for beloved people she has not seen for many years.

The news of the cancer had an interesting effect on Nana:

almost as though she had been waiting to know what would bring about her eventual death, she seemed so relaxed that several family members wondered whether she had really understood the news. But this is the wisdom of a long life: none of us is immortal, and every day brings us closer to our last. In her eighties, Nana had a stroke that affected her use of language. She lost words, and substituted others in ways that sometimes made her speech impenetrable, and on other occasions was unintentionally wildly comical. Her mobility became limited too. She accepted these burdens with determined stoicism. In retrospect, I suppose she expected that another, fatal stroke would rescue her from living a limited life, but here she is more than a decade later, still talking to us about sausages and 'You know, that . . . whatever . . .' with a roll of the eyes that says, 'Mm-hm! You know *exactly* what I mean!' while we cast around for ways in which 'sausages and something else' might be relevant to the conversation about, for example, her new duvet cover or what she would like to send her great-niece for her new baby.

So now she knows. Not another stroke, but cancer. Painful pressure on her pelvic nerves has been giving her a pain 'down there' (rolls eyes) that she didn't like to mention. She has been losing weight, and off her dinners a bit, but not enough to cause any alarm. When the palliative care team's recommendations for the nerve-compression pain are effective, she is quietly pleased. 'That was like a . . .' – rolls eyes – 'a . . .' – eyes indicate 'down there' – 'Polaroid,' she explains, and while my aunt looks perplexed, my sister remains heroically straight-faced as she says, 'Yes, Nan, like a haemorrhoid.' The rest of us rummage in bags and pockets to avoid catching each other's eyes and creasing with inappropriate laughter.

So, because I am here and I may not get another chance, I am in the watching rota. Last night I slept in my childhood bedroom in my parents' house, and no one was on watch because Nana seemed comfortable and rested. But today, suddenly, she has begun to change. Sleepy and awake by turns; too weary to eat; accepting occasional sips of fluid; asking for the Pope. The priest came to visit; she was delighted. Fancy the Pope coming so quickly! Goodness knows how that conversation went, but she seemed very peaceful afterwards.

By evening it was clear that, her burdens laid down, Nana was preparing to die. A visitor from her nursing home, a diminutive and very experienced nursing nun, spotted the signs and asked her where she wanted to spend her last days – no beating about the bush. Nana wanted to 'get home', and the knee-high nun said they would expect her home tomorrow. The ward staff agreed to make the transfer arrangements. Nana smiled and slept and slipped into a coma. All things I have seen many, many times, yet never really *seen* at all.

And that is how I come to be perched on the edge of this chair in the darkness, searching the face and the sounds of my frail and failing grandmother. Suddenly she opens her eyes and says, 'You should be . . . not here . . . asleep . . .' Almost a sensible sentence. I touch her cheek, and notice that her nose is cool at the tip.

'Nana, you have walked the floor at night for all of us. Now it's our turn. Just sleep. I'm comfy here, and it's lovely to be with you . . .' And she smiles, a gummy benediction of a smile that brings tears to my eyes. 'Mum and Auntie have gone for a cup of tea. They'll be back soon. Can I get you anything?'

She shakes her head and closes her eyes. From out of nowhere, the sound of Brahms' lullaby floats into my mind, its halting waltz-time reinterpreted as a bedtime lullaby sung to each of her thirteen grandchildren in our turn (and probably to our parents before us, too) in Nana's deep, cracked yet soothing voice. Here, at the edge of her dying, I contemplate the meagre understanding I have of her long and often troubled life, and the intimate knowledge that she has of mine. She is a remarkable woman, yet I hardly know her. She modelled self-reliance and resilience to my mother and her siblings, and to her eight granddaughters and five grandsons.

Before she became unable to converse with fluency, she was a confidante of our woes and transgressions, an adviser in anxieties and a source of solace in times of trouble. She knows us inside-out, but she said so little about herself; and we self-absorbed youngsters never thought to ask.

How many people attending a deathbed must realise these truths, as they see a future they had taken for granted slipping away from them, a much-loved person slowly descending through the layers of consciousness towards coma and death? No wonder there are fantasies about swansongs, in which people linger for a last word, a deep revelation, a declaration that all will be well.

Nana's breathing is soft now, panting and shallow. How many times have I described periodic breathing to families, to medical students, to patients themselves? And yet, it never sounded like this before. This sounds like someone who has run a long way, who is breathless, who is anxious. But her face is serene, her brow unfurrowed, and her pulse (I feel her wrist) is steady, regular and sedate – and I notice that, like her nose, her hand is cold. I tuck it beneath the crocheted shawl Auntie brought from home earlier today, as though in some way I can warm it into life. My professional self is satisfied that she is not in distress, yet I am poised and alert, like a security officer guarding an at-risk target. All my senses are primed to spot the least disquiet.

The shallow breathing pauses. I hold my own breath – *Oh no, please don't die when they've gone for a tea break.* And then she takes a huge, snorey breath, and that other pattern of periodic breathing begins, slow and deep and noisy. I think of the number of times families have asked me if the sound indicates distress, and I have wondered why they mistake snoring for intentional vocalisation; yet here I am, listening intently for any suggestion of an edge of perturbation to that well-known, sonorous boom of a snore that kept me awake at night whenever she came to stay when I was a child. Slowly, as I know it will, this automatic breathing gets faster and shallower, and then so shallow that I can't hear it, while I scan every breath, and watch her face, and search for any suggestion of a waggling toe or a tiny hand movement that may suggest that she is trying to make contact one last time.

The next twenty minutes pass in this way before Mum and Auntie reappear with a paper cup of orange hospital tea for me. I feel as though I have been alone here for an eternity, watching and evaluating my comatose grandmother, searching for meanings and discarding them again. We are past the point of communicating; the loss weighs like a heavy stone in my chest. I offer to stay the night, but Auntie will not hear of it – the night shift is hers, and tomorrow I have a long train journey back to my small children and my busy job and my kind husband. I know that I will not see Nana again.

In fact, getting home perked Nana up immensely, and we did see her the next weekend, propped up on pillows, pale and diminished yet delighted to see us all. Between long snoozes she enjoyed short conversations.

I was not there when she gave the last out-breath the following week. But I had learned the lessons of the vigil, and through the kindness of the natural order – watching a grandparent's death. Since then there have been other vigils, with the same intensity of active watching and exhausting focus, and with sadness at the untimeliness of deaths before their right time (as though there is a right time), but also with recognition and appreciation of the last lesson I learned at my grandmother's knee.

Now that I understand how minutely attentive to detail the watchers are, how active and probing their attention is, how exhausting the responsibility feels, I am a better servant to their needs and questions, and so much more patient with their frequent requests to check for any sign of discomfort or distress. This last vigil is a place of accountability, a dawning realisation of the true value of the life that is about to end; a place of watching and listening; a time to contemplate what connects us, and how the approaching separation will change our own lives forever.

How intently we serve, who only sit and wait.

Pause for Thought: Patterns

The stories in this section have been chosen to illustrate the gradual, predictable sequence of events as we die that used to be familiar before medicine progressed and dying at home became more unusual. Knowing what to expect is immensely comforting to the dying person and their supporters. Once we all know what we need to know, we can relax with each other. It's surprising how relaxed a well-prepared family can be around a deathbed.

Have you ever been with somebody while they died? How does what you saw match the patterns described in these stories? Is the description of dying what you were expecting? In what ways does this information affect your view about the experience of dying? How well do you think TV dramas, soaps and films deal with dying and death? Do they help us to be better prepared, or does drama displace reality?

When you are dying, where would you like to be? What are the pros and cons of being at home in your own bed (perhaps moved to a more accessible room), or staying with a relative or friend, or in hospital, or in a care home, or in a hospice?

If you have seen a death that appeared uncomfortable or shocking, how have you dealt with that memory? What information in what you have read in this section could allow you to re-evaluate what you experienced?

If you regularly have upsetting memories of a difficult situation, whether it is a death or something else, and especially if the experience still feels as though it is happening again there and then, this suggests that your experience may be causing post-traumatic stress disorder (PTSD). Your doctor can help. Please don't suffer more than you need to – ask for advice. There are some useful suggestions in the Resources section at the end of this book.

My Way

Human beings are highly resilient. We adapt to adversity, and find ways to maintain our inner peace as best we can. Often, we use coping patterns that we developed very early in life: if you've always 'put on a brave face', then that becomes your preferred way, and you may find it difficult to understand someone who copes by sharing their distress out loud. Neither you nor the other person is coping better or being braver than the other; one simply finds inner peace by venting, whereas the other's peace comes from feeling self-contained. If you are a 'take control and plan the details' person, it can be tough for both of you if you are sharing a distressing situation with a person who copes by thinking about everything *except* the challenge ahead: one person's avoidance is in direct conflict with the other's need to plan, and this is stressful for both of them. Finding middle ground on which to meet and work together requires sensitivity, tact and patience, and perhaps even the help of a trusted third party.

The next few stories offer some insights into the widely different strategies people use, often completely spontaneously and without any insight into their own behaviour. You may recognise types of people you know very well – you may even recognise your own style.

Everybody prefers to manage things 'my way'. The end of life is no different.

That is the Question. . .

The strength of the human spirit is astonishing. People all think that they have a limit, beyond which they cannot endure. Their capacity to adapt and to reset their limits has been a constant wonder to me over my decades in working with people living with some of the most challenging illnesses imaginable.

Eric was a Head Teacher. With capital letters. He was an organiser, a man who Got Things Done. He managed a large inner-city comprehensive school, and 'his kids' knew that he would support them through any challenge, whether by telephoning the deans of their university faculties or by attending their interviews under caution at police stations.

Being a head teacher demands a lot of one's time. Over his career, Eric (and his family) had made this sacrifice, and he was looking forward to spending much more time with his children and grandchildren when he retired. Developing motor neurone disease was not part of his plan.

His illness presented itself slowly. He caught his toes from time to time while running on a treadmill, but when he fell off the treadmill completely, his GP found some odd reflexes in his legs and sent Eric to hospital to check he hadn't damaged his back. The spinal surgeons said his back was fine, but he had three years or less to live. Those 'odd reflexes' and occasional trips were the first signs of a creeping paralysis of all his muscles as they gradually lost their instructions from the nerves that connect them to the spine and brain. This is MND.

Remember, Eric was a head teacher: he got things done.

Naturally, he looked up his illness on the internet. The news, delivered on screen, in writing and with no pacing or pauses for thought, was horrifying. Eric decided that he would kill himself before he became a burden to his wife. He considered a variety of ways to do this. Should he fake an accident by driving into a motorway bridge support? Or could he use tablets? Perhaps a plastic bag? He got more information from the internet, and tried to imagine how and when he should act.

Faking an accident seemed his best plan, and he aimed to kill himself before the grandchildren could notice his illness. He hated the idea that they might consider him decrepit. If he accomplished his mission before the summer, then he judged that everyone would recover in time to take a special holiday at Christmas that he had booked, with gleeful anticipation, when he retired. Eric had a plan and a timeline. On a bright spring morning he set off in his car 'to collect a parcel from the post office', with the secret intention of killing himself. The next thing his wife knew was when he walked back into the house just a few minutes later and said, 'I can't manage the gearstick.' Paralysis of his arms had begun, and his driving days were over. So much for Plan A.

Spring became summer, and Eric gradually lost the use of his arms and legs. He had an electric wheelchair that he used in the house and around the local streets. He played with his grandsons, who were thrilled with his wheelchair and covered it with Batmobile stickers. He was astonished that they were not at all daunted by his increasing immobility, and loved straightening his spectacles or helping him to blow his nose. Carers helped his wife to get him up and dressed in the mornings and back into bed at night; his daughter who lived nearby came with her sons after school each day to give her mother a chance to go shopping. Eric realised that committing suicide with tablets (Plan B) was likely to be impossible now that he was never alone.

So Eric, who had been a Head Teacher who Got Things Done,

was now a man in a wheelchair who had things done to him. He had expected that he would hate this, that he would be a burden, and that he would rage against the indignity of immobility. But to his surprise, he found that he was still a man who could Get Things Done. The vegetable garden he had planned was tended by his wife and son, with Eric nearby as adviser ('That's not a weed, it's a row of parsnips, you turnip!'), and they relished their outdoor time together. He designed a pot garden for herbs beside the kitchen door, and it was planted by his grandsons under his supervision. He played chess, read books, savoured a fine single malt.

Eric's wife, Grace, was a great cook, and relishing his meals became Eric's daily pleasure. By the summer, though, even this was a lengthy chore as the task of chewing and swallowing became more difficult. Along with eating problems, Eric had increasing difficulty with speech as his lips and tongue became weaker. He knew from his internet research that some people with his condition needed feeding tubes to keep them nourished. He decided that he would rather be dead than not eat 'the way nature intended', and wondered whether he could starve himself to death. This became Eric's Plan C, although he didn't yet have a start date.

At midsummer, Eric developed a new problem. In effect, he had delicious-dinner-related pneumonia, because his swallowing muscles no longer protected the top of his windpipe. Some of that lovingly prepared soft food had been silently sliding down into his lungs when he swallowed. He wondered about letting himself die of his chest infection, but because he was hot, breathless and uncomfortable he opted to have treatment. He was admitted to hospital for intravenous antibiotics.

I first met Eric that week. He wasn't sure the palliative care team had anything to offer him. Weren't we a bit useless? He explained his absolute opposition to a feeding tube. He explained his hope of an early death so that the family could recover and have a happy Christmas. He explained his belief that euthanasia would be a good treatment for him, and his frustration that it was forbidden by law. He explained his decision to stop eating as soon as he was sent home from hospital.

It was clear that this was a man who Got Things Done. If he decided to starve himself, he would succeed. So we discussed what help he might need to remain as comfortable and as in-charge as possible while he was dying. He said that he feared pressure ulcers on his skin (very sore and possibly smelly), and seeing his family in distress. And choking – he was pretty certain that his illness would end in an episode of choking. Taking his concerns one by one, we considered ways to address them.

Pressure ulcers are sores that break the skin open, usually where it is squeezed and stretched between a bone on the inside of the body and furniture or clothing on the outside. They can be very painful (think how much a single blister hurts in a tight shoe), and become more likely as a person loses the ability to shift their position on their mattress, and as they have less fat padding their skin. So Eric was right – I agreed that he was a sitting duck for pressure ulcers. This unfortunate pun was the first glimmer of humour in our relationship. His eyes twinkled and his lips twitched, and he gave a wheezy, weak laugh.

Potential ways to avoid pressure ulcers, I suggested, might be to keep him rotating on a rotisserie-type gadget not yet invented for humans, or to avoid malnutrition.

'But,' he countered, 'if I avoid malnutrition, then I won't be killing myself, will I?' Movement of eyebrows suggests he has categorised me as 'stupid as well as useless'.

'Anyway,' he continued, 'if I eat, I'll choke.'

'So let's think about choking,' I say. 'What do you mean by choking, exactly?'

The eyebrows are starting to look a bit cross, but he explains with great patience, as though I am a particularly dim pupil, that he means *choking* – when something gets stuck in your throat, and blocks it, and you can't get it out, and you can't breathe, and you die horribly in front of the very people you have dedicated your life to protecting . . . Tears suddenly spill down his cheeks.

And there it was, the very nub of Eric's distress: not choking, in fact, but failure to fulfil his mission to protect. He protected the children of so many other families throughout his career, yet now he feels unable to protect his own. He can't even induce his own death to safeguard their peace of mind.

'And it will be awful for them, and you can't bear to do that to them?' I suggest, dabbing his tears and wiping a drip at the tip of his nose. He nods and holds my gaze with his. 'And how have they responded to choking episodes so far?' I ask. He considers, and tells me that he hasn't had any – yet.

'Why do you think that is?' I say. 'Just good luck? Soft food? Or what?'

'Well, I'm still waiting for that to start,' he says. 'Or rather, I want to die before it starts.'

'So if I were to tell you that people with MND do not choke as a terminal event,' I say, 'what would you make of that?'

'I'd ask you for your evidence. Prove it!'

I have evidence. There is a palliative care survey of several hundred MND patients, followed up until they died, and precisely none of them died by choking. 'That's not to say that they didn't have occasional episodes when they struggled to clear the phlegm in their throats – and it's hard to clear your throat when your cough is very weak, isn't it?' He nods. 'But nobody died choking, and nobody's family had to watch them choke to death. Dying is gentler than that. Shall I describe what they are likely to see?'

Concentrating carefully, he allows me to tell him what we see as people die. 'That's amazing,' he muses slowly. 'That's just amazing. So it's safe for me to swallow?'

'Well, actually no, it's not safe,' I remind him. 'Because some of the food goes down the wrong way, and that will damage your lungs. But if you don't mind the lung damage, and you want the pleasure of eating, then I'd say you have a choice.'

He is still listening intently; we are now collaborating, where initially I felt we had been debating.

'And I would say you have more choice than that, too. If you want to avoid pressure ulcers, you could have that feeding tube put through your skin straight into your stomach, to have liquid-ised meals without the bother of trying to chew and swallow every calorie. And if you decide to stop using it later on, that is your right.'

Eric, the man who Gets Things Done, has some thinking to do. I leave him to ponder. The following week, I hear that he is to have a feeding ('PEG') tube inserted, and will be going home once Grace has learned how to give the feeds. And there our acquaintance might have ended, had it not been for Christmas.

At home, he used the feeding tube for all his nutrition, but swallowed very small amounts of delicious food created by Grace, just for the pleasure of eating. He often had a coughing spasm after swallowing, but considered this a price worth paying. When he developed another chest infection, he declined to go to hospital but agreed to come to the hospice, where once again he was given the choice of whether to have the chest infection treated, and once again he opted for antibiotics.

His mood was low. He told one of the nurses that he felt that he was a burden to Grace, and that he wished he could die. Despite this, he wanted to live until Christmas. This was a surprising contradiction, and the nurse explored it. Eric thought that there was now insufficient time for his family to recover from his death before Christmas, even if he died in the next few days. Accepting antibiotics was part of his new plan to control the timing of his death. All his plans to shorten his life had failed, so now he was trying to prolong it instead.

The nurse asked about the Christmas deadline, and the full extent of Eric's love of family time at Christmas poured out: the gathering, the gifts, the rituals about particular decorations on the tree, the songs, the family stories with new embellishments each year. It was a time when they were thankful for each other, for their family life. Eric wanted that Christmas experience, for himself and for all of them, just one last time.

On the ward round the nurse repeated this conversation, and the team pondered the dilemma. Eric was unlikely to live beyond mid-November: the muscles in his chest were becoming weaker, his breathing at night-time was beginning to fail, and he had decided that he would not use a ventilator to assist his breathing. He was running out of options. *If only Christmas were closer. . .*

When we proposed moving Christmas, Eric grinned. 'There will have to be a tree . . .' he said.

It was a joy to see that tree, the table set with linen, china and glasses, the stockings along the hospice window ledge. On a windy autumn evening the family arrived in Christmas jumpers and fancy clothes, carrying gifts and musical instruments. Their host greeted them at the front door of the building in his bed, pushed by two nurses wearing Santa hats, who delivered him, along with his oxygen cylinder and tubing, into the training room the catering team had set up like a five-star restaurant. Off-duty staff in formal dress waited on the family; turkey and trimmings were served; Eric's oxygen was turned off briefly so the pudding could make a glorious, flaming entrance. After dinner, those of us on duty could hear guitars, Christmas carols and lots of laughter coming from the party.

Two days later, Eric sent for me. He told me that he wanted to stop his antibiotics. 'I'm ready to die,' he said, 'and this is my chance. I'm glad I didn't kill myself earlier. It would have been too soon, I would have missed so much. I had no idea that I would be able to tolerate living such a changed life.'

He closed his eyes. Thinking that he was tired, I got up to leave. He commanded me to sit down and listen. 'This is important,' he said. 'People need to understand this. *You* need to understand this. I wanted to die before something happened that I couldn't bear. But I didn't die, and the thing I dreaded happened.

But I found that I could bear it. I wanted euthanasia, and no one could do it. But if they had, then when would I have asked for it? Chances are I would have asked too soon, and I would have missed Christmas. So I'm glad you couldn't do it. I've changed my mind, and I wanted to tell you. I was angry with you because you're part of the System that says no to assisting with dying. But you weren't saying no to dying, you were saying yes to living. I get that now. I'm a teacher, and you need to tell other people this for me, because I won't be here to tell them.'

And then I was dismissed from the head teacher's presence.

In fact Eric's pneumonia was improving, but he was becoming very weak. The day after this conversation, he was too sleepy to talk. A day later, he was unconscious. Surrounded by his family, and with a Christmas tree in the corner of his room, he died gently and without any hint of choking, after that last wonderful Christmas.

Never Let Me Go

Denial is an effective psychological mechanism for dealing with distressing situations. By choosing not to believe the bad or dreaded thing is happening, a person can avoid distress completely. Difficulties may arise as it becomes harder and harder for them to ignore evidence that something is seriously wrong: if they have not accepted any bad news at all, then nor have they made any emotional adjustment for it. If their denial breaks down suddenly, they may become completely overwhelmed by the realisation of how bad things really are.

For families, it can be a huge challenge to live alongside someone who is maintaining denial of an unpalatable truth.

How should we respond as professionals when there is no time left to adjust? Is complying with denial telling lies, or respecting the person's choice?

In a single hospice room filled with postcards, furnished with her own cushions and fabrics from home, an enfeebled young woman with a vibrant mane of red hair is pacing. Supported by her mother, she lowers herself carefully to sit on a brightly coloured blanket that has been placed on the chair. Her husband and her father look on warily from the small sofa bed. She strokes the softly brushed wool, and a stream of babbling words pours from her lips. 'Feel how *soft* it is! It's alpaca. Remember when your brother came back from Peru with it, Andy? When I'm better, we're going to Peru with him; he knows all the best places to visit. I want to see those temples to the sun. The god has huge hair. He looks like me! I could be the sun-god . . .'

She cannot settle. Rising to her feet, and almost falling as her swollen right leg fails to do her bidding, she bats away the anxious attention of her mother and limps back to the bed, perching on the edge. She faces the sofa, where her father and Andy are sitting in silence.

'Cheer up, you two!' she commands. 'Nobody's dead!' She coughs and sighs. This is Sally, and she is dying. But nobody can mention it.

Nicola, one of the nurses, enters the room, bringing Sally's medications: drugs to prevent pain, nausea and breathlessness caused by the cancer that is tearing through her body.

'Ah, cocktails!' beams Sally with a brittle smile, and Nicola pours her a glass of water. Sally takes the glass, but her arm cannot take its weight, and the water spills on her clothes, on the bed and on the nurse. 'Drat it!' she shouts, suddenly angry. 'Why did that happen? I'm soaked! Don't just look at me like that' – to the men. 'Go and get a towel! No, Mum, I *don't* want another one. For heaven's sake, WHY ARE YOU PEOPLE ALL SO USELESS?!' She bursts into tears.

Nicola observes Sally's restlessness, her weakness, her outburst of anger, the flood of tears. She wonders whether, despite her efforts to ignore the rapid deterioration in her health, Sally is starting to sense that all is not well. Using denial to cope with an unbearable sorrow can help someone to avoid facing their distress, but if they can no longer maintain their defence, the cataclysmic truth can rush in like an unstoppable tide, drowning them in their own dread. Nicola suspects that, after several years of staunch denial, Sally at last senses the oncoming torrent. Wisely, she deals with the spilled glass rather than the tide of terror, then returns to the office for help.

I had known Sally since her cancer was first diagnosed. Then she was a party girl, a redhead with a sumptuous fountain of burnished copper hair, a glowing, shimmering radiance cascading around her shoulders; a Pre-Raphaelite goddess. And this is relevant, because chemotherapy makes people's hair fall out.

I first met her while I was a research fellow in the cancer centre, taking on a research project for the Professor of Oncology as part of my palliative medicine training; Sally's party dancing was impeded by having had her right big toe amputated to stop the spread of a melanoma that had been found growing underneath her painful toenail. She told me that she was 'going to fight it' when I arrived to put up her drip; she was too busy enjoying life to let cancer get in her way. She had Plans.

'Tell me about your plans,' I encouraged her as I swabbed her arm and prepared to insert the plastic cannula through which she would have a chemotherapy drip for the next few hours.

She gathered up her flowing, curly halo of hair with her free hand to keep it away from my work, then took a breath, smiled, and said, 'Well, I want to learn to windsurf. Somewhere warm. Greece, maybe.' Her eyes took on a faraway gaze. 'You can go on watersports holidays and get taught to do all kinds of stuff. And then I want to go to Australia and visit the Great Barrier Reef and learn to scuba-dive. It's supposed to be amazing!' Then, leaning forward, she peered at the cannula now sticking out of her arm and said, 'Have you done it already? I was expecting something bigger, and lots of pain and blood and stuff!'

As I taped in the cannula and attached the saline drip, waiting for the chemotherapy bag to arrive from the hospital pharmacy, she carried on explaining her plans. She seemed simply to say aloud whatever was passing through her mind.

'I want to travel,' she said. 'I want great holidays. I want to marry Andy. And we'll have an amazing honeymoon somewhere really fantastic, like the Himalayas or the Alps. He loves climbing. But he hates water. We're like chalk and cheese! It's like that "opposites attract" thing, you know? I mean, he's so quiet and thoughtful and clever, and I'm like, "Wheee! Look at me!" and he's like, "I'm trying to concentrate here, do you mind?" with his head in a book or watching some film about climbing or nature and stuff. I don't know how we'll make it work, but we will. And I'll learn to cook and make all his favourite meals and I'll learn to be quiet – shhh – yeah, like' – *whispering now* – 'so quiet when he's thinking about things.'

She cannot maintain the whisper, and launches on, apparently exuberant and enthusiastic – or is she terrified and garrulous? It's so hard to tell. 'But obviously I can't be a bride with like no hair and that, so we'll have to wait until my hair grows back after the drugs, but it's worth it to be cured and I'll look back on all this when I'm an old lady and all this will seem like a crazy dream. I'll beat this. I know I will.'

I am caught up by her enthusiasm, so it is only later in the day, while grabbing a sandwich with my colleagues during a teaching session, that I consider the vital role of our big toe in balance. Windsurfing and climbing will be extremely challenging without a big toe. And do you need a big toe to flap a flipper when you're diving? I waggle my outstretched foot thoughtfully, until the speaker meets my eye and I realise I have not heard a word of the lecture. Sally is occupying my mind, chattering and disturbing my concentration from the other side of the hospital.

Three weeks later, she is back for her next round of chemotherapy. I almost don't recognise her: without her tumble of hair she is delicate and pixie-like, her features naked without eyebrows or lashes. She greets me enthusiastically with another stream-of-consciousness monologue. 'Hi, doc! Here we go again! Oh boy, I was so sick after you left last time. Can you give me anything extra for the sickness? It's just the worst. I hope I never get morning sickness. I mean, can you imagine feeling like that, but for *months*?! Un-be-liev-a-ble! I want lots of kids. Andy's blond, so we might have more ginger-nuts like me. I think ginger babies look soooo cute, don't you?'

I explain that I will not be putting her drip up until I have checked that her bone marrow and kidneys have recovered from the previous round of chemotherapy; I will take a blood test now, and get back to her as soon as I get the results. She looks disappointed. 'Just bring it on!' she announces. 'I need to get better, so get that cancer-poison dripping!' While I prepare my needle and tubes for her blood test, I ask her to tell me what other plans she has for her future life with Andy. She says she wants 'at least four kids', and she has ideas for their names already; the blood is in the tubes before she stops talking and blinks, eyes owl-like in her round, bare face. 'Crikey! I never felt a thing again!'

Actually, she is so distracted by her own ideas and plans that she simply doesn't notice the jab of the needle. It's not due to any skill on my part – it's her own coping device, the power of her mind in action, to behave almost as though we are pals meeting for a coffee and catching up on all our news: 'Nothing wrong here . . .'

This week her drip is put up by one of the chemotherapy nurses, so I don't see her again until I am leaving for home. She is sitting in the car park, drip still running, having a cigarette with a tall, angular man with short fair hair and round-framed spectacles. 'Hey, doc! This is Andy. Andy, this is the Professor's assistant. She's the chief poisoner.'

I walk across the car park to say hello. I learn that Sally just has to wait for a bag of saline to run through ('It's rinsing my kidneys. I *know* it's doing me good!'), and then Andy will take her home. He looks tired and anxious. In fact, *he* looks like the sick person; if Sally were not bald and towing a drip stand, she would look completely well.

Over the next four months, Sally continued to attend for her chemotherapy every three weeks. She vomited profusely, but always came up smiling and imagining how other people must be having a worse time than she was. She had steroid tablets to reduce her nausea, and these gave her plump, pink cheeks. She looked radiant. Andy, meanwhile, became increasingly gaunt and haunted-looking. I almost expected to see him with his own drip stand.

And then Sally's treatment was over. The research nurses saw her occasionally in the Professor's clinic, and reported that she was well. We got a postcard from Greece (*'Hiya Poison Team. Said I'd do it so here we are. Can't stand up on a wind-surfer but kayaking is brilliant!!! Keep up the great work. Sally'n'Andy xxx'*). I lost touch with her progress when I went back to work at the hospice at the end of my research project, but I often thought of her when I met patients who coped with their misfortune by making little of it and thinking about how much worse things were for other people. Her denial had supported her through the ordeal of her treatment.

Since then, two years have passed. Sally's hospice referral took me by surprise, because I didn't recognise her married name. The plastic surgery ward team had asked for advice about managing a young woman with widespread melanoma. There was some concern that she didn't seem to realise how serious things were, and they wondered whether this was due to brain secondaries or to a psychological problem manifesting as denial. I was sent to assess her by the leader.

On the plastic surgery ward, the doctor explained that their young patient had devastatingly widespread melanoma and a life expectancy of just a few weeks. Her groin was completely encased in the cancer, which was growing outwards through the surgical wound where removal of the affected lymph nodes had been attempted. Back-pressure from the groin tumour was causing her whole leg to swell. She had multiple lung nodules, getting bigger week by week on her X-rays, and also liver deposits that were almost certainly growing at a similar rate. 'And yet,' he sighed, 'she seems not to hear any of this bad news when we tell her. She just tells us it's an infection in her wound, and that chemotherapy will cure her. I've never come across anything like this. We just don't know how to handle her.' He invited me to walk down the ward with him, to be introduced to the patient.

I saw that unforgettable hair shining across the hospital ward, and recognised her before she realised who I was. Her face was swollen by high-dose steroids for her headaches; she had a compression stocking on her right leg and the remaining four toes on that foot, swollen, shiny and disconcertingly purple, stuck out of the elasticated cuff. Pale and thin beside her sat Andy, disintegrating like Dorian Gray's portrait while she beamed at me with an inner splendour despite her ruinous disease.

'Well, doc! Long time, no see! What a surprise!'

It is to me, too, I thought apprehensively.

'Well, it's been a busy time since I saw you last,' she announced. 'Look! Andy and I got married!' She held up her left hand for me to inspect her engagement and wedding rings, a rather splendid interlocking arrangement of jewellery clearly made specifically for her. *So you did achieve that plan.* I was relieved that she had accomplished some of her dream in time.

'Bit of a hiccup with the melanoma thing, though,' she continued breezily. 'I got a few lymph nodes in my groin and there's a bit of melanoma in them, so I might need a little dose of chemotherapy. But there's an infection in the wound. And you *know*' – she grinned conspiratorially at me – 'that they *never* give chemo when there's a bug on board, so I'm waiting for the infection to clear first. It's making my leg swell a bit. But I'll beat this. You know I always do. Have you come to see me about the chemo?'

She paused to draw breath. Andy looked at me with wide-eyed anxiety, and the ward doctor also watched my face, clearly wondering how I intended to tackle this situation.

This was exactly the same coping style Sally had used of old: downplay the negatives, emphasise the tiniest positives, pretend it will all be fine, make plans for the future. She seemed unaware of her true situation, but a single glance at Andy told me that he was fully alert both to the devastation that was unfolding, and to his wife's inability to contemplate it.

What will happen if I say 'Hospice?' I wondered. *Will she find an excuse? Will she be shocked? Will she dismiss me? Will all her denial come crashing down around her? How on earth do I play this?*

'Well, congratulations on your wedding,' I began. 'It seems like a lot has happened to both of us since we last met. You've got married, and I've changed careers . . .'

'Aren't you a doctor any more?' she asked, surprised.

'I'm a different sort of doctor now. Good old Professor Lewis is still trying to find the cure, and I hope he does, but in the meantime I'm trying to get to grips with tricky symptoms like headaches and nausea and breathlessness. Things that make people feel unwell.'

'Well, I have ALL those symptoms!' she almost squealed – perhaps disinhibited by her steroids, or by nervousness as I brushed too close to her own problems.

'Then maybe I'm the right doctor for you just now,' I said. Andy's head nodded gently in agreement behind her; the ward doctor dashed away to answer his pager.

When I asked her what she believed the current problem was, she replied, confidently and without hesitation, 'It's all down to this infection.'

'Do you ever worry, even for a fraction of a second, that it could be something more serious than that?' I asked her gently. *Oh, this feels like very thin ice . . .*

'Of course not – I have Plans!' was her immediate, calm response. 'I will get better. I will beat this. I mean, I'm not *stupid*. I know there's cancer in there. It's just that as soon as the infection has gone, I'll have chemo and *beat* the cancer. Because it's time we had those little redheaded babies. I'm not getting any younger! And neither is Andy.' She reached out, took his hand, and squeezed it reassuringly. 'I'll be *fine* once I have the chemo.' Andy bit his trembling lip.

So, this was complete denial. I had read about it. I had discussed it with our liaison psychiatrist. But I had never before met denial as rock-solid as this. In the face of overwhelming disease and week-by-week deterioration in her health, Sally had found an alternative explanation that allowed her to maintain perfect equanimity, even optimism.

Over a series of cautiously phrased statements, I explained to
Sally that I work in a place that specialises in symptom management, and that some of our patients just come for a while to be
made well enough for further treatment. I was about to go on to
say that others are sick enough to die, but she interrupted me.

'That's what I need!' she declared. 'I need to get well enough
to come back here for my chemo. Where do you work, then?'

Gulp. I'm going to have to say it.

'Have you heard of the hospice?' I asked her.

She smiled. 'Yeah! They looked after Andy's gran last year. They
were fab. Do you like it there?'

'I love it. It's a great team. And I know they would love to help
you. Fewer headaches. Less breathlessness. How would you feel
about coming across this week?'

I can't believe she's remaining so calm.

'It sounds ideal,' she said. 'It's much easier parking. Andy can
come for longer, and my parents can visit more easily too. And
then, when you've made me feel better, I can come back for my
chemo.'

So, two weeks ago Sally came to our hospice for symptom
management, hoping every day to become well enough for further
chemotherapy whilst every day becoming weaker, slower, more
limited by breathlessness. We were able to maintain her physical
comfort, but her emotional distress was barricaded behind the
walls of denial that she maintained despite all the evidence. Until
today.

Entering Sally's room, Nicola, another nurse and I find Sally
in restless motion. Her mum has helped her to change her T-shirt;
the men have gone through the French windows onto the patio
outside, where Andy is smoking a cigarette. Sally rubs her hands,
licks her lips, rubs her eyebrow, gathers and drops and regathers
her hair. As she does so, she speaks constantly. 'I just need a bit
of fresh air. I don't want you to turn the light out. Mum? Mum!
Stay here. Where's Andy? When will this infection get better? I

want to get home but there's too many stairs. Howdy, hello girls'
– to us. 'Did you see I tried to drown Nicola? Sorry about that!
Are you drying out?'

Nicola holds a glass of water and helps Sally to take her evening
medications while the other nurse and I change the wet bed. Then
the two nurses expertly guide their weary patient onto the clean,
dry sheet, plump up her pillows, adjust the headrest, and there
she is, sitting up with her painful leg supported on cushions and
her auburn halo scattered across the pillows.

'Sally, what's happening?' I ask her, taking a seat on the arm
of her bedside chair so that our eyes are level.

'Same as ever,' she says. 'Waiting to be ready for my chemo.'

'How's your breathing?' I ask, noting that she is panting slightly.

'All right. I get a bit breathless when I feel impatient. But that's
normal, right?'

No, it's not normal. But she doesn't want to hear that.

This is a tricky situation. Sally seems agitated and anxious, yet
she declines to admit even to the idea of that anxiety. We have
all (except Sally herself) noticed that she has been far more sleepy
for several days, taking daytime naps with ever-decreasing levels
of energy in between. The staff have recognised that she is beginning the process of dying, but she absolutely does not want to
discuss any outcome other than getting well enough for chemo,
having babies and living happily ever after with Andy. Today she
can barely hold a glass of water. Her anxiety is driving restlessness
that uses up what little energy she has, and her fear is fighting
the slow creep of unconsciousness. We have drugs that can take
the edge off her anxiety, but I am aware that by reversing her
distress, we may allow her to drift into dying.

I also know that she is exhausted, agitated and unable to relax.
I know that a small dose of sedative will relieve this exhausting
agitation, but I am unable to ask Sally for informed consent
because she cannot, will not, accept the facts of the situation. I
decide to give a tiny test dose of the anti-anxiety drug, and to

plan our next move when we see whether or not it reduces her agitated restlessness.

We chat as we wait for the half-tablet to dissolve under her tongue.

'Sally, how are your energy levels today?' I ask, wondering whether she has observed the changes in herself.

'Oh, not great. But I have a lot of sleep to catch up on from when the pain was bad. I do keep dozing off . . . Could it be the morphine, do you think?' She shuffles her position and begins restlessly gathering and dropping her hair again.

'Well, morphine sometimes makes people a bit woozy for the first few days, but you've been on this dose for two weeks, and it wasn't making you sleepy before. So I don't think it's the morphine. I think it's more likely that you're a bit less well –' (*testing . . .*) 'and needing a bit more sleep.' *Will she pick up that cue?*

'Well, when do you think I can start that chemo? My pain is better and my nausea has gone, so things are definitely getting better. I'm going to beat this cancer, you know.' *No, she is not taking the cue. Denial still solid. What astonishing self-protection!*

I am not prepared to storm her defences and leave her open to the full realisation that death is now very, very close. Somehow, our team will need to work with Sally's family to manage her dying while preserving her denial. And, of course, this means that there will be no chance to say goodbye.

I ask Sally's permission to talk to her family in a quiet room down the corridor.

'They can talk here!' she proclaims.

'Of course they can,' I agree, 'but in my experience, lots of families feel better if they can talk to the doctor in private. They can get stuff off their chests. Please may I take them away? Nicola will stay here with you while we talk.'

'Well, I'll want a full report when you all get back!' says Sally. But I know she will find a way of avoiding that report.

I take the family to a quiet room around the corner, where

they confess to each other that they think Sally is dying, and I confirm their suspicions.

'Do you think she realises?' asks her mum, tearfully.

'What do you think?' I ask.

She twists a handkerchief around her fingers as she looks searchingly at her husband. He shakes his head and looks at Andy. Andy looks at the floor. There is a silence. Then Sally's mum says, 'She knows, but she doesn't want to talk about it.'

The men stare at her, and I encourage her to say more.

'Sally can't bear it. She can't bear the sadness. She can't bear the fear. She can't bear us to be sad. So she's looking the other way. And we have to help her to keep pretending.' She looks pointedly at her husband and says, 'Her dad thinks we should be honest with her. But I think we'll break her if we do that.'

Andy looks up, gazing into the middle distance somewhere, and says, 'I agree. It's like when I'm doing an extreme climb. Part of my mind knows that if I fall, I'll die. But thinking about the danger will only make it more frightening, and more dangerous. I need to focus on the rock, on my grip, on my feet, on the wind, on the rope – everything except the danger. That's what she's doing now, focusing on everything else . . .'

'Andy, that's genius,' I exhale with relief. He understands, and his metaphor can carry the family through this challenge. 'It's as though we are all supporting her to keep her focus on what will help her most, and that is staying calm. So we can be truthful' – her mum looks startled – 'but not with the whole truth.'

To explain further, I suggest that they can truthfully tell her how much they love her, how proud of her they are, what memories from her life so far they treasure, what kindnesses of hers they have appreciated. These are all parts of the Last Messages that we observe around many deathbeds, and yet they are not Goodbye.

'And if she wants to talk about a future we cannot see,' I continue, 'then we will simply encourage her. She has names for her unborn children' – her mum sobs loudly, and is consoled by a gently patted shoulder, which is all her husband can reach – 'and plans for future holidays. If they help her not to look at reality, then we will just allow her to choose where to focus. Can we all support that?'

Everyone nods. We head back to Sally's room. She is now sitting in her chair, and is clearly less restless, although she looks a little bit more sleepy. She doesn't ask us what we talked about. Andy has captured her dilemma perfectly, and the whole family is on-script. Nicola and I leave the room, and Sally says, 'See you tomorrow, doc!'

When I arrive in the morning, Nicola meets me on the corridor to tell me that Sally's glorious sun has finally set. She was still planning to beat this thing as she lapsed into unconsciousness.

Hat

People are not limited so much by their illness as by their attitude to it. The illness may present physical challenges, but the emotional challenge is often far more important. Our human spirit may stumble as the path ahead appears too daunting, yet with support and encouragement, our resilience can be re-enabled and used to find creative solutions. We are all individuals, and one person's plan may not be a good fit for another who, outwardly at least, appears to be in a similar situation. Enabling people to be architects of their own solution is key to respecting their dignity. They are only in a new phase of life; they have not abdicated personhood.

Penny was choosing a wedding dress in a rather refined shop with her mum, Louisa. As she reached out to straighten Penny's veil, Louisa felt her hipbone snap with a loud crack. She went very white and passed out on the powder-pink carpet, and there was a flurry of ladylike panic as the *grandes dames* of the trousseau tried to ensure that their prostrate customer didn't crush any dresses. They also thoughtfully rang for an ambulance, so by that evening Louisa was in an orthopaedic ward with her leg immobilised and a diagnosis of cancer secondaries in her hip, from a breast cancer treated several years previously. Penny hadn't chosen a wedding dress either.

Louisa did not thrive on her orthopaedic ward. In the late 1980s a broken hip was initially managed by holding the broken bones in position using a series of weights and pulleys to pull against the strong muscles that anchor our legs to our pelvis, because if the thighbone breaks, those same muscles unhelpfully pull the bone shards painfully into the soft tissues of the thigh. Fit, young patients with sports or trauma injuries might then be offered a hip replacement, but cancer patients would be offered radiotherapy and weeks of immobility to see whether the bone would reunite to allow walking again.

Louisa realised that she would have to spend her daughter's wedding day in hospital, in a nightie, with her leg suspended in mid-air. This is not a traditional look in wedding photographs. She was devastated, and missing the wedding was worse news than knowing that her cancer was back, and was now incurable. She pined, declined, lost weight, wept, and descended into a deep, intractable depression. Fitter patients with hip injuries came in for surgery and left walking with crutches, while Louisa stopped colouring her hair and let her grey roots start to show, lost interest in make-up or even discussions of wedding dresses, and adopted a helpless, hopeless gaze. The nursing team, affected by her hopeless helplessness, reduced their contact time as their attempts at cheery banter were rebuffed. Louisa became an isolated, lonely and frightened statue.

Millie was a childminder whose most recent employers no longer needed childcare. She was relieved; she was sixty years old, and feeling more like ninety. Her left hip ached at night and clicked as she walked, hurrying after children made her breathless, and Millie decided that her working days were over. She lived alone, socialising with her many friends from the local Nigerian community with whom she swapped stories of home and compared recipes with 'work arounds' using British ingredients to cook the soul food of her home country. One of her friends noticed that Millie was limping, and advised her to see a doctor. Millie didn't like doctors. 'They tell you that you are ill,' she protested, 'then they suggest all sorts of treatments. Ever since I arrived in England, I have avoided doctors. That is why I have been so healthy!' Despite having lived in England for forty years, Millie retained her lilting

Nigerian accent, and she accompanied her declaration with a
throaty, contagious laugh.

In fact, Millie was avoiding doctors because she had a weeping
sore on her right breast, and she was embarrassed about it. She
bathed it and dressed it twice a day, but it was becoming bigger.
She was a single lady, a tidy and careful person, and she thought
a doctor might think that she was not clean. It was only when,
with a loud bang, her hipbone snapped while she was choosing
hair oil in the city's 'Nigerian supermarket' that she was forced to
see a doctor by being conveyed to the hospital, with many of the
other customers in support, by the shop owner's son in their
delivery van. Millie's X-rays showed that not only was her hip
broken, but many cancer deposits were dotted about her other
bones. Suspecting a possible breast cancer, the casualty department
doctor examined her for lumps. She found the dressing and, after
gentle persuasion, Millie revealed her shame.

'Oh, Mrs Akonawe, this must be so sore for you!' said the
doctor, and Millie immediately felt safe. This kind lady knows I
am clean, she realised, and now she will help me.

Responding to the doctor's calm questions, Millie described
how the ulcer had begun more than two years previously as a tiny
lump. 'I thought it was an insect bite,' she said, 'but it just got
bigger and then opened up.' The doctor examined Millie's armpit,
found hard, swollen glands, and asked whether her arm had become
swollen. 'My fingers swelled so that I had to remove my mother's
wedding ring,' replied Millie, 'and I wear it now on a chain. My
skin feels thick down that arm. I do not know why.'

The doctor explained to Millie that the ulcer might be something serious, and that the arm swelling was because whatever was
causing the ulcer was also blocking the lymph glands under her
arm. Millie was perplexed – what could this serious thing be? The
doctor asked her about her energy levels, and Millie described
how tired childminding had made her. 'I could hardly keep up
with those children! And when their mother took them home, I

just fell asleep. I did not want to visit friends because I was so tired. Sometimes I did not even cook.'

The doctor summarised their conversation, and as she did so, Millie began to see a pattern, a downward, frightening pattern. Reducing energy, breathlessness on exertion, a weeping ulcer, a swollen arm, painful legs, a sore hip. 'Doctor, please tell me – do you think I have HIV-AIDS?' she asked. The doctor was surprised; she had thought she was leading gradually to telling Millie about cancer. She had not anticipated this diversion.

'Mrs Akonawe, do you worry about HIV? How do you think you might have caught HIV? Do you have a husband?'

Millie shook her head.

'Forgive my intrusive question, but when did you last have sex with a man?'

Millie pursed her lips in surprise, and exclaimed, 'Never, doctor! I am a virgin woman, an unclaimed treasure. I left a fiancé in Nigeria when my father brought us here, and I have never loved anyone else!'

The doctor squeezed Millie's hand, and nodded before saying, 'Another way people catch HIV can be from a blood transfusion. Have you ever had a blood transfusion?'

Millie shook her head. 'Doctor, I have never been ill or had any treatment ever! I am proud of my fitness. Or I was . . . but now, I do not feel so fit. No, indeed, I do not.'

'Well,' said the doctor, 'the other way people can catch HIV is by sharing needles for drugs. Do you use injected drugs, ever?'

Millie smiled. 'Doctor, I can see you are teasing me, because you know that I am not That Kind of Woman. You mean, my illness is not AIDS?'

The doctor nodded, but added, 'Not AIDS, but still something very serious.'

Millie blinked. The doctor explained that her symptoms could all be explained by a breast cancer, starting in her ulcer, spreading to cause pain in her bones, swelling in her arm, and breathlessness.

The cancer-weakened hipbone had then given way. Her hip was broken, and she would need several weeks in bed. Millie silently absorbed that information. 'Will I die?' she asked, after a long silence.

The doctor said, 'We need to find out whether this is cancer, and what sort of treatment would help you to get better. We'll admit you to the orthopaedic ward, and they'll strap up your leg and arrange more tests.'

And so it came to pass. Millie was admitted to the orthopaedic ward with a broken left hip, and found herself in a bed next to a pale, withdrawn woman with a broken right hip – Louisa.

The Nigerian supermarket crew brought 'proper' food in for Millie that evening, and Penny found there was something of a party atmosphere at the women's end of the ward when she arrived with photos of the wedding dresses she had shortlisted to show her mum. Louisa simply wept, but Millie's visitors spotted the wedding dress photos and immediately began to offer advice.

'Look at you, so beautiful!' said Millie's next-door neighbour. 'Big blue eyes and . . . yes, you get them from your mummy, anyone can see that. Millie, look, don't these women have identical, beautiful eyes? You look more like sisters!'

'What a beautiful bride you will be!'

'I hope you are marrying a good man!'

'What happiness! What a wonderful day you will have!'

Louisa listened as these kind women give Penny the sort of talking-up every bride should get from her family, and she felt her heart break – like a physical snapping inside her chest, as she realised that she was now only a burden, and her illness, her brokenness, her misery, were all spoiling Penny's joy. After visiting time, she turned her face to her pillow and wept for all her lost expectations. The night nurses discovered her weeping, and the following day they rang the hospice for advice. The leader did a ward visit, and proposed to Louisa that she might find her bed rest more pleasant at the hospice. Transfer was arranged.

Whilst awaiting transfer, Louisa became ever more withdrawn and sad. Beside her, Millie held court and offered deep-fried plantain slices to the other ladies – a real hit. Visiting times were colourful and vibrant, with Nigerian food and loud prayers being celebrated around Millie's bed. By now, Millie's breast cancer had been confirmed, and both she and Louisa were wheeled downstairs for radiotherapy to their broken hipbones every day. Millie seemed surprisingly joyous. She was hugely relieved that she 'only had cancer' after her fear of AIDS. She had also started tablets that were reducing the size of her ulcer and the swelling in her arm, and she had never been so tenderly looked after in her adult life. Hospital seemed like a good start to her retirement.

Penny was gratified when her mum settled into the hospice and allowed a psychiatrist to visit her. Treatment for her depression began, a combination of a new 'talking treatment' called cognitive behaviour therapy (CBT), and some tablets that had made her sleepy, so she declined to continue them. The CBT challenged some of her hopelessness, and encouraged her to try mini-experiments to check whether or not her feeling of helplessness was actually justi-fied. Cautiously, she began to re-engage with daily activities: she agreed to let a hospice volunteer give her a manicure, and loved the restoration of her hands with bright nail polish. She asked the hairdresser to retouch her roots. She asked Penny to bring in her make-up bag. She even asked for her bed to be wheeled into the garden so she could watch the birds. It was there that she smelled deep-fried plantain and heard Nigerian music coming from another bedroom, and so discovered that Millie was also in the hospice.

Millie was delighted when Louisa asked to be allowed to visit her. Millie's hip pain had not settled well after her radiotherapy, and she had been transferred to the hospice for pain management. She was in a single room, and felt lonely. Louisa was wheeled along in her bed, and they discussed recipes, the contrast between hospital and hospice, their collapses in shops when their hips broke, Penny's wedding, and Louisa's sadness that she was going to miss it – and then Millie had an idea.

'The day after you left the hospital, a young doctor come to see me and he aks me if I want to join an experiment. He aks me if I want a new hip joint to take away my pain. But I feel too old, I tell him thank you and no thank you. He tells me his team is finding out if putting in a new hip is a good treatment for cancer. Why don' you find out if that could work for you? Those girls on that ward, they was walking on their new hips, wasn't they? An' if you could walk, you could jus' glide down that aisle with your beautiful daughter . . .'

Millie did excellent public relations for the orthopaedic department's clinical trial, and the next day an excited Louisa asked the nurses whether she could have surgery for her hip. The leader gave me the job of asking the orthopaedic team, who had not offered Louisa a place in the trial because her mood was too low for her to engage with the consenting process. When they heard that she was keen, a research nurse and doctor were with us within an hour, and less than three weeks after she had arrived at the hospice, Louisa was on her way back to the hospital for surgery. It was a gamble, but with her immaculate hair and shining nails, she was ready to fight. Her experiments with CBT had restored her sense of purpose.

One week later, Louisa arrived back at the hospice with a new hip and a lot of stitches. Instead of lying in a bed, with ropes and pulleys attached to her leg, she arrived in a wheelchair followed by Penny, holding a walking frame. 'You can hide *that* thing,' Louisa told her. 'I am *not* being seen with a walking frame!'

Louisa and Millie were now in adjacent beds in a four-bedded bay, and Millie's pain was settling. They were both visited by the physiotherapist each day, Millie for exercises to keep her good leg supple, and Louisa to begin the task of walking on her new hip joint. Louisa kept up a stream of distracting chat while Millie carried out her uncomfortable exercises, then Millie acted as a

commentator as Louisa gained command of elbow crutches, and
then her (much despised) walking frame, taking just a few steps
initially, until she could raise herself to a standing position from
a chair, and walk across the bedroom as far as the bathroom door.

The hospice receptionist popped her head into the bay. 'Louisa,
there's a couple of parcels for you,' she announced. Louisa turned
pink.

'What have you done, girl? You look tickled!' shouted Millie.

Louisa smiled a sidewise grin, and said, 'You just wait!' to her
friend before asking for the parcels to be brought to the room.
And what parcels! There was a cardboard box the size of a cricket
kitbag, and a huge cylindrical hatbox. Sitting in an armchair, and
using her bed as a table, Louisa set to, pulling tapes and tearing
ties until her packages were open.

As we staff gathered to admire, a dark pink dress, a cream
jacket, a silky cream-and-pink chiffon shawl, brand-new underwear, and a small box were produced out of the larger parcel. In
the cylinder nestled a hat fit for Ascot Ladies' Day, cream with
dark pink trim, at least half a metre wide and utterly exquisite.

'What's in the little box, Louisa?' asked the physio.

'You won't approve . . .' said Louisa as she withdrew a pair of
dainty, low-heeled cream sandals, 'but this is our next target. I need
to be able to walk down the aisle in these shoes in three weeks'
time. And nobody tell Penny! This is our secret, my big surprise.'

The physio shook her head, smiling. There's nothing like a
motivated patient.

The tradition is that a bride is married from her parents' home,
so a hospice single bedroom was made available as Penny's dressing
room on her wedding day. She was coming to the hospice straight
from her hairdresser, and Louisa was going to help with her
make-up and supervise her dressing in her gown and veil, aided
by her two bridesmaids. Penny believed that her mum would be
attending the wedding in a wheelchair with a nurse escort, so

Louisa met her from her taxi in a wheelchair, already resplendent in her pink and cream finery, although not yet hatted.

'Wow, Mum, you look wonderful! How on earth did you shop for all that?'

Louisa smiled. Before she had collapsed in the wedding-dress shop, she had been discussing mother-of-the-bride outfits with one of the *grandes dames*. While Penny was being scooped into a particularly complex white meringue by a *dame* with a mouthful of pins, Louisa had fallen in love with this raspberry and cream affair, and had determined to try it on later. Later, of course, she was somewhat preoccupied with pain, pulleys and palaver as her wedding-day planning was crushed by cancer. It was only when the Nigerian ladies had modelled wedding enthusiasm in the orthopaedic ward that Louisa suddenly realised how far she had abandoned Penny, and how wide the gulf had become.

Part of Louisa's CBT work with the hospice's visiting psychiatrist had been to contemplate ways in which that gulf might be bridged. Step by step, working towards a goal of 'giving Penny all my love and support on her wedding day', Louisa had begun by writing a speech to be read in her absence by a relative at the reception. She then visited the church with our physio, to discover that there was wheelchair access, so she would be able to attend the ceremony. This triggered a phone call to the *grandes dames*, who of course would never forget those particular customers, to ask if they could supply the coveted outfit, and add 'a hat and shawl big enough to hide a wheelchair' – in which quest they had succeeded beyond her dreams. The idea of inviting Penny to dress at the hospice was another of those plans. With each step Louisa became more engaged in the wedding and in Penny's planning. Her mood began to lift and her ambition to soar, a virtuous circle of engagement, planning, pain management and love.

The bride and her mother emerged from the bedroom, with two bridesmaids in attendance. Penny's simple, elegant ivory dress and trailing veil were set off to perfection by her radiant smile as she and her bridesmaids wheeled Louisa (well, Louisa's hat – we couldn't see Louisa) up the corridor towards reception. In the day room, a guard of honour of two rows of patients ranked in beds, wheelchairs and armchairs, attended by staff with cameras and hankies, applauded the wedding party to the door. Millie and the Nigerian ladies wept and sang, clapping and swaying to a wedding song from home. At the door, the mother of the bride asked her attendant to stop. The physio produced that walking frame, now decorated with the chiffon shawl, and Louisa rose to her feet. Nodding her majestic millinery, and smiling like a child at the funfair, Louisa walked her astonished daughter to the waiting limousine, to escort her to her wedding.

What about 'happily ever after'?

Louisa was able to return to her home, living on the ground floor, after some further advice and innovative furniture placement by the hospice physiotherapy and occupational therapy experts. She was tired after the wedding, and began to discover that she no longer had the energy she was used to. As a single parent, she had always assumed that Penny's marriage would open up possibilities for her own retirement, but now she found that she was limited to short bursts of activity, like walking to her local shop or a day out at hospice day care. She always popped in to see Millie on her weekly day-care visit, and she made a tour of the hospice with the wedding photographs. Louisa noticed that Millie was looking pale ('Not an easy thing to spot!' laughed Millie), and that she was often snoozing at the start of Louisa's visits.

Millie became more quiet after Louisa went home, and asked her visitors to come only in pairs to avoid exhausting her. The radiotherapy took effect so that she no longer needed the traction apparatus attached to her leg, and this allowed her to sit in a chair and be wheeled around the hospice gardens. Her appetite began to fail – even plantain crisps were no longer relished. Gradually, in continuing parallel, the two friends became weary.

Two months after the wedding, Louisa developed pain in her other hip. X-rays showed thinning of the bone caused by another cancer deposit. Millie was beginning to lose her breath if she tried to talk too quickly, as the cancer deposits reduced the efficiency of her lungs. Despite these trials, every day she thanked her God that she did not have AIDS. Louisa was readmitted to the hospice for pain management and bed rest. The partnership was restored.

Louisa died three months after Penny's wedding day, and Millie the following week. With similar ages and almost identical tumour burdens, these sisters-in-arms had chosen very different ways to adapt to the challenge of a broken hip. Millie's stoic acceptance of bed rest and traction had enabled her to live an engaged and outward-looking life despite her limited physical horizons. Louisa's courage had demonstrated to the orthopaedic team the profound benefits of hip replacement, even in the last year of someone's life.

Hip replacement is now the treatment of choice for people with hip fracture caused by cancer. Much credit must be given to those early orthopaedic surgery pioneers, and to the lady in the cream hat.

Louisa's rapid response to CBT was astonishing, and it piqued my interest in this patient-empowering approach to managing emotional distress. A few years later I was to train as a cognitive behaviour therapist, and to discover the satisfaction of using CBT to enable palliative care patients to rediscover their inner resilience, to challenge their unhelpful thoughts and to take steps towards coping again in a life still to be lived, despite their advancing physical illness.

Take My Breath Away

Being a cognitive therapist as well as a palliative physician has enriched my practice. Outside the calm of the CBT clinic, though, during busy hospital ward consultations or at appropriate moments during a hospice ward round, opportunities would arise to use a CBT approach in a simpler way, to help a patient (or the clinical team) to gain more insight into a knotty problem.

This led to referrals from hospital colleagues for a 'CBT first aid' approach to anxiety, panic and other overwhelming emotional distress.

Whether CBT first aid or the full CBT intervention, the core principle is that we are made unhappy by the way we interpret events. Distressing emotions are triggered by disturbing underlying thoughts, and helping a patient to notice these thoughts and to consider whether or not they are accurate and helpful is key to enabling them to change.

'I'm not talking to a shrink,' Mark greets me. It is Boxing Day on a respiratory ward. He is leaning forward, legs crossed and elbows protruding, all skin and bone, like a stick insect in an oxygen mask. His T-shirt, clinging to his sweaty chest, shows his protruding ribs and the suck of the muscles between the ribs with each panting breath he takes. This is a man on the edge – of what? Terror, anger, despair?

'Lucky I'm not a shrink, then,' I reply.

He surveys me gravely. 'They said you mess with people's minds.'

'It doesn't look like your mind needs messing with,' I say, and he rolls his eyes. 'But your mouth is dry, isn't it? And so is mine. Shall we have a cuppa?'

We negotiate. If I prove to be capable of producing a decent cup of coffee ('Five sugars, cream if there is any . . .') then he will agree to talk to me, provided there is no 'messing with his mind'. And if he says stop, I will stop. Leaving his door ajar, I make for the ward kitchen (just past the seasonal chocolate mountain) and discover the high-quality coffees and gourmet teas that have been given by grateful relatives for Christmas. *Even squirty cream. Providential.*

How do we come to be here, when both Mark and I should be in our own homes celebrating Christmas? It's like this. After several years of running a CBT clinic for palliative care patients, I began to see some recurring patterns. This was useful in applying a 'CBT first aid' approach while working in a busy hospital palliative care consultation service, away from the peace and protected time of the clinic. Among the patterns is the very human response of fear in the face of breathlessness. This is primal, a survival instinct (we talk about people 'fighting for breath') and an important reflex in saving us from environmental dangers like drowning, choking or smoke inhalation. However, that same reflex drives an exhausting battle when the breathlessness is caused by a life-threatening illness damaging our respiratory systems. Then, accepting some breathlessness and struggling less would make for more comfortable living towards the end of life.

One of the patient groups where I frequently met troublesome breathlessness was young adults with cystic fibrosis. This is an inherited condition that gradually damages the lungs, pancreas and digestive system during childhood and teens, often leading to death before the age of thirty. A few patients survive longer thanks to improved management of damaging chest infections, and better remedies for their diabetes and nutrition problems. Some may survive long-term if they are lucky enough to have a successful lung transplant. Timing of lung transplantation is critical – it is a high-risk procedure, and so should be delayed while the patient can manage a reasonable quality of life, but not to the point that the patient's deteriorating lungs make them too ill to survive the anaesthetic and the surgical procedure. Our hospital palliative care team works closely with the cystic fibrosis team, offering advice to reduce the impact of breathlessness, cough, gut problems and weight loss, whether as palliative measures or to prepare people to be fit for surgery. We also work psychologically with a few patients whose anxiety and panic generate increased breathlessness.

When my home phone rang on Boxing Day, I was surprised to hear the voice of a respiratory physician at the hospital. He was calling for advice about a twenty-two-year-old man with cystic fibrosis. Mark had end-stage disease. His only hope of survival was a lung transplant. He was clearly a resilient guy: over the past fifteen years he had coped with gradually progressive breathlessness, but had continued his education, played and later supported football, been part of a group of 'lads' who enjoyed drinking beer and making jokes. He had not let breathlessness stop him. Yet for the last five days he had been sitting bolt upright in bed in a hospital room, in terror. He could not be left alone. He could not bear the door to be closed. He was panting into an oxygen mask, despite not really needing oxygen therapy. Five days previously he had seen the transplant surgery team, who had told him that he was now a candidate for transplantation. He had been given a radio pager so he could be contacted day or night if organs became available. Although nothing else had changed, he had changed his view of his survival chances over the thirty minutes of that surgical consultation. He was too frightened to go home after his clinic visit.

'Can you come and see him?' asked my colleague, adding, 'How soon can you get here?'

It's Boxing Day!

I called a taxi.

The nursing team greeted me warmly and took me straight to

Mark's room. He was sitting like a castaway on his hospital bed island, a tower of pillows behind him instead of a palm tree, wide-eyed and staring over a hissing oxygen mask. A physiotherapist who was sitting anxiously beside him darted for the door, murmuring, 'Mind if I leave you to it?' as he slid rapidly out of the room.

Once I had passed the coffee test, our conversation could begin. Mark described the sensation of working hard to breathe, associated with dry mouth, heart palpitations and a sudden realisation that he was about to die, that had gripped him at least three times an hour since he had been given the radio pager. Although conversation was handicapped by Mark's hissing mask and his penchant for expletives, we were able to draw out his experience as a sequence of steps, as follows:

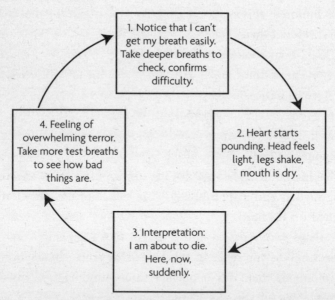

1. Notice that I can't get my breath easily. Take deeper breaths to check, confirms difficulty.

2. Heart starts pounding. Head feels light, legs shake, mouth is dry.

3. Interpretation: I am about to die. Here, now, suddenly.

4. Feeling of overwhelming terror. Take more test breaths to see how bad things are.

Mark was intrigued. As I drew the experiences he was describing into the diagram, he leaned forward to watch, even though this constricted his chest movement. He became irritated by the hissing of the oxygen mask, and moved it from his nose and mouth to the top of his head, where it was held in position by its elastic thread, like a tiny policeman's helmet. He began to point out the sequence of events, and to add details, until he was satisfied that the model described what he was experiencing.

'What do you make of that?' I asked him. He pondered. He took the paper and pen, and emphasised the arrows. He underlined the word 'terror'.

'It's a vicious circle,' he declared. *Absolutely.*

'So, let's just consider for a moment,' I suggested, 'because that experience looks really horrible. I'm not surprised you can't sleep or be left on your own. How many times has that happened to you now?'

Together, we calculated that it had happened at least three times an hour, at least twenty hours a day (because he dozed off occasionally at night), for the past five days. That added up to around three hundred episodes of feeling he was about to die at any second. How exhausting.

'OK,' I invited him to reflect. 'You've felt on the brink of death three hundred times in the last few days?' He agreed. 'And how many times have you actually died?'

He blinked at me and shook his head.

'Well, how many times has the resuscitation team come in to save you?' I asked.

Shaking his head, he regarded me suspiciously. There was something vaguely and inappropriately comical about the oxygen mask perched on his head.

'Perhaps you've passed out?' I asked. No, apparently not.

'So what do you make of this belief that you're about to die at any moment, then? It's happened three hundred times, and it hasn't yet caused you to collapse, faint or die . . .'

There was a long pause. He took a deep breath, then exhaled slowly and in quite a controlled way. We had been talking for forty-five minutes. *He isn't using the oxygen. And he hasn't missed it. Time to test out a theory . . .*

'It's probably time I asked why you're wearing your mask on top of your head,' I said. He started, dropped the piece of paper and grabbed the mask, suddenly breathing rapidly and with his eyes rolling in terror. I held the diagram in front of him and asked where in the vicious circle he found himself. He jabbed a finger at 'terror', and continued to pant. I asked him why he thought he needed the oxygen now, when he had worn the mask on his head for more than thirty minutes without missing it at all.

'When you feel ready, Mark, I wonder whether you could lift the mask away from your nose again,' I said, while he panted and swore with astonishing fluency inside the mask. Gradually the heaving of his chest slowed. Cautiously, he raised the mask off his nose and removed the elastic from around his head, so he could hold the mask in his right hand while picking up the diagram with his left. He grinned at me tentatively.

'It's panic, isn't it?' he said.

Bingo. He's absolutely right. Got it in one.

Together we examined his belief that he might die at any moment, and considered other possible explanations for his terrifying experience. He remembered the 'flight or fight' response from long-ago biology lessons in school; the way the body makes adrenalin to deal with any threat, causing deeper breathing, faster heart rate and tense, prepared muscles, primed with oxygen and ready to take action to save our lives. He could also describe the physical sensations he experienced when his beloved football team was awarded a penalty at a critical point in an important game. As the player places the ball on the penalty spot and walks back before taking the vital kick, many people can describe the physical symptoms of adrenalin release: dry mouth, pounding heart, breathlessness, weak legs, sweaty palms . . . yet we describe this experience as 'excitement'. Wedding-day nerves can feel the same, but brides don't generally interpret them as a fear of impending death.

We began to modify our diagram, as Mark understood the role of adrenalin and the sense of anxiety that was giving him more symptoms, and his mistaken but understandable assumption that the symptoms caused by adrenalin were a danger to him.

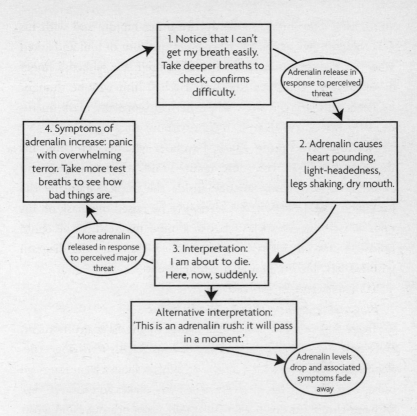

Before leaving, I asked Mark if he thought he could explain this diagram to his dad, who had been waiting outside the room. And could he please have some more panic attacks so he could check out our hypothesis, and add any symptoms we might have missed. He grinned and agreed.

This is cognitive therapy for panic. The model is usually used when otherwise healthy people misinterpret innocent physical sensations of adrenalin release, but it is just as relevant, and can be incredibly helpful, for people who have real breathlessness and whose focus on their symptoms prevents them from engaging in anything else, in particular in anything pleasant. This is a conversation Mark and I will have next time we meet.

Two days later we are reviewing his diagram and his experiences of the past forty-eight hours. Predictably, now that he understands the mechanism of the adrenalin–heart pounding–terror link he has had only five more episodes of panic, and one of those was triggered by 'thinking about that gorgeous nurse'. *Sense of humour is returning. Good sign.*

Mark still believes he is too fragile to manage at home, but he has contemplated the 'oxygen on the head' episode, and has realised that he was not breathless while we were drawing the diagram because he was completely distracted. We make a list of distractions he could use in hospital to deal with breathlessness. He agrees to use these to see if he can manage to get out of his room and go to the lift block; and possibly go down in a lift to the coffee bar. Particularly if *that* nurse could be his escort.

The expedition to the lift block is a success. The next day, Mark and a physiotherapist go down in a lift to the coffee bar; he enjoys himself so much that he is away for half an hour, and the ward send out a search party. Amused, he puts on warm clothes and crosses the road to the park. And then goes into town for a half day with his pals.

On my first official day back at work, I greet the new year by visiting Mark in his room. He is delighted with himself. He has been to the pub with friends, and nearly got into a fight. How? Well, apparently he is using a different set of distraction techniques when he is out of his room, ranging from innocently looking at makes of cars, to more provocatively looking for ladders in women's tights, and estimating their bra sizes (which was what nearly caused the fight).

Mark did get home. We continued to meet for CBT, and he managed his breathlessness by using distraction and remembering non-threatening explanations for his symptoms. This worked for three months, but with no lung transplant available he developed another chest infection that tipped him back into hospital.

The ward team phoned me on a Saturday to say that Mark was dying, and did I want to see him. *Does he want me to? Yes. Are his parents there? Yes.* Come and check there isn't anything we're missing, they said.

I was glad to go. Mark's favourite physio had also come in on her day off, and was in his room along with Mark's parents and the ward sister. All were solemn and red-eyed. Goodbye is always hard.

'Oh, it's you,' he greeted me, lying in a foetal position propped up by pillows, and with oxygen pipes up his nose. He was breathing very fast, and was only able to say one or two words per breath. 'Are you here for coggy thingy or pally whatsit?'

'I'm here to see if you need a decent cup of coffee,' I said. He grinned, then asked his parents to leave the room for a moment. His glittering eyes shifted around the room, vigilant and wary, yet his smile was sincere.

'You should be fucking proud of me!' he announced, his ability to swear still utterly intact.

'Really? Why's that then?' *I am not going to cry.*

'Well, look at me. I'm fucking dying, and I'm not fucking panicking!' he declared, delighted with himself and allowing himself a deathbed swagger.

Smiling tearfully at each other (*OK, so perhaps I am going to cry*), we both understood that this was Mark's great moment of personal triumph. He realised he was dying. He was about to be given drugs to relieve his breathlessness that he knew would also make him sleepy. He had already told his mum that he couldn't bear to see her being sad, so she must wait outside and his dad would keep watch while he was dying.

Using CBT principles that he had been practising for only a few weeks, Mark had managed his distress, planned his deathbed, and as he said, he was not panicking. He had learned not to fear his fear, and he guarded his peace of mind heroically to the last.

This episode of care had many repercussions. The ward team used Mark's diagram to understand his panic and to talk him through it, instead of giving him unnecessary oxygen and making him dependent on reassurance. The cystic fibrosis team saw the benefit of a psychological intervention even at the very end of life, and a member of their nursing team trained as a cognitive therapist and has gone on to produce a transformational clinical service and groundbreaking research on the impact of CBT-based support for people with respiratory diseases. Breathlessness is terrifying: CBT helps people to understand and manage their terror, instead of feeling controlled and undermined by it.

The success of a psychological intervention lies in how far the patient moves from unhelpful beliefs, thoughts and behaviours to new and more helpful ones, and therapy is most helpful when the patient perceives that they, and not the therapist, are the agent of change. This could be regarded as 'not getting the credit', but in fact it is perhaps the most rewarding outcome of all to watch someone fly high and proud on their own, because therapy has given them wings.

Pause for Thought: My Way

These stories have shown different ways in which people cope with difficulties: trying to keep control; avoiding the truth; sinking into helplessness; simply accepting whatever fate has in store; using resilience to adapt to events; and becoming anxiously preoccupied with the threat of the situation. Which of these patterns do you recognise in yourself? You may have more than one style.

Which coping styles do you recognise in the people closest to you? How might your individual styles make things easier or more difficult for each other if you had to deal with a challenge together? How could you have a conversation now to acknowledge each other's styles?

Each of these coping styles has positives as well as negatives – for example, helplessness has the attribute of allowing others to help, which can be a struggle for people with some of the other styles. So remember to look for each other's strengths and resilience, as well as any potential 'flashpoints'.

If you worry about having a conversation like this with someone you know well, then perhaps you could join in a 'death café', either on your own or with your loved one. These are friendly, informal gatherings at which people can mull over various aspects of death and dying over a comforting warm drink and excellent cake. There are death café meetings in more than forty countries, and they always welcome new visitors.

Naming Death

It has become taboo to mention dying. This has been a gradual transition, and since we have lost familiarity with the process, we are now also losing the vocabulary that describes it. Euphemisms like 'passed' or 'lost' have replaced 'died' and 'dead'. Illness has become a 'battle', and sick people, treatments and outcomes are described in metaphors of warfare. No matter that a life was well-lived, that an individual was contented with their achievements and satisfied by their lifetime's tally of rich experiences: at the end of their life they will be described as having 'lost their battle', rather than simply having died.

Reclaiming the language of illness and dying enables us to have simple, unambiguous conversations about death. Allowing each other to discuss dying, rather than treating the D-words as magic ciphers that may cause harm merely by being spoken aloud, can support a dying person in anticipating the last part of their living, in planning ahead in order to prepare their loved ones for bereavement, and can bring the notion of death as the thing that happens at the end of every life back into the realm of the normal. Open discussion reduces superstition and fear, and allows us to be honest with each other at a time when pretence and well-intentioned lies can separate us, wasting time that is very precious.

Second-Hand News

Communication through conversation between two people is such an intrinsic part of life that we often take it for granted, yet we are all aware of occasions when friends and family get hold of the wrong end of the stick. What they thought they heard us say is not, in fact, what we thought we meant. Now multiply the possibilities of mis-hearing, misunderstanding and getting lost in translation when a person gets important news from their doctor, and then tries to report it back to their family afterwards. It's a recipe for disaster.

Early in my career, I had the good fortune to be offered a twelve-month contract as a cancer research fellow, working in an academic cancer centre with a prestigious and groundbreaking team. My role was to see patients in clinics and on the wards who had agreed to take part in trials of new drugs; sometimes these were anti-cancer drugs, and sometimes other medications intended to reduce the side-effects of treatment. Over the year, I was mainly dealing with patients for whom no possible options for cure remained, and who knew that their only treatment options were aimed at improving their quality of life or possibly extending it by a short time. Some of these patients bravely offered to test new anti-cancer drugs, aware that they were unlikely to experience any personal benefit yet willing to help our research in order to contribute knowledge that might help future patients. For some it was a personal anti-cancer crusade; for others it was making sense of their impossible situation by using their misfortune to improve other people's fortunes in the future; for some it was a form of bargaining with God or the

Fates, in the hope that their reward would be an unexpected improvement in their own health.

I saw most of these patients very regularly. In addition to their admission for two or three days' treatment with new chemotherapy agents every three weeks, I saw them weekly to take blood tests that monitored the impact of the drugs on their body, and to ask them about any side-effects they were experiencing. We talked about other things too, of course: how they were managing, what their families were up to, what plans they were making for Passover or Eid, the progress of a daughter's pregnancy or a grandson's apprenticeship application. They probably spoke to me more often than to their friends and neighbours, and I certainly saw more of them than I did of my own family.

In this way I got to know Fergus. He was a stocky, gruff-voiced Scotsman who had worked as a shepherd on his uncle's farm from the age of eighteen. He loved the hills, the wide sky and the endless vistas. He was a quiet, shy man who confessed that he had been too timid to talk to girls as a youth, and had anticipated that he would be 'married to the farm'. He was completely unprepared for the shock of falling in love at forty-three with the woman who managed the stock pens in his local meat market. He was captivated, and too mesmerised even to remember to be bashful. Within eighteen months they were married and parents to a son. Five years later Fergus was my patient, gently turning yellow as an aggressive cancer relentlessly replaced his liver.

Fergus joined in a study of a new drug for his type of cancer. 'I have tae beat the bastard thing,' he said. 'I have too much to live fer. My Maggie, my lovely girl, how can I leave her when I've only just found her? And the Boy . . .' His eyes would lock onto my face, searching for some sign that I had good news, that I might be offering recovery, some respite, some extra time for his unlooked for, unexpected, joyous family life. He always called his son 'the Boy'. He said it reverently, as though he was talking about something too sacred to be named.

His fourth course of the treatment was due in mid-February, just before the Boy's sixth birthday, which fell on Valentine's Day. Fergus would be home in time for the big day, but the treatment always left him wretched, gagging and puking for five days before he could fall into a sweaty, forty-eight-hour sleep that restored his ability to talk to his family again. He came for his blood test the week before. He had been into town, and he showed me a beautiful locket he had bought for Maggie as a Valentine's gift. 'I'm going tae put a photo of the Boy on this side,' he said, 'so he'll be at the front. And she likes this old photo of me, see' – producing a snap taken at a family wedding in which he is young, broad and strong, with a mop of dark curls, and strong legs below his smart dress kilt, laughing and raising his dark brows above eyes creased from the weathered horizon-searching of his trade – 'so I'll cut the head oot and put it in the back. That way, I'll always be right close tae her skin. Always. Whatever happens.'

I asked about their plans for the birthday. They would be at home, he told me, just the three of them together. 'We've bought the Boy a bike, just wee with stabilisers. It's blue. He has no idea. He'll be so tickled . . .' Fergus's eyes lit up at the thought. I knew that his liver scan was not improving, and that postponing his treatment for a week, to avoid the birthday being wrecked by his resulting nausea and exhaustion, would make no difference to his overall outlook. He was losing ground; gradually more yellow, starting to look gaunt.

'Fergus, how will you be over the birthday if we go ahead with the treatment next week?' I asked. 'Will you be able to enjoy the bike, the cake, the event?'

'Och, I'll prob'ly feel crap, I always dae, you know, fer a few days at least. But I cannae give up!' Defiant lift of the chin.

'What if we delay the treatment by one week? That won't be giving up. It would let you enjoy the birthday, and Valentine's Day. And then you can come back for the next treatment afterwards. A few days off won't make a difference. What do you think?'

He considers, knitting his deep, thoughtful brow. 'It wouldnae do nae harm to put it off fer a few days?' he asks tentatively.

'I don't think so. Do you want to talk it over with your wife?' I ask. I know she is in the waiting room, but he had left her there and come into the clinic room alone. 'I can talk to her now, with you, if you like.'

'No, nae need to bother wi' that,' he says. 'I can explain. Aye, let's bide a wee bit. I might be able to help wi' the bike that way.' He smiles. 'Important family time, birthdays, eh? I have great memories o' mine when I was wee. I want that fer the Boy.' He picks up his jacket. 'So, back to the ward on 19th then, is it? Or dae you need a blood test next week?' I tell him the 19th will be fine. 'Thanks then, doc,' he says. 'See you after, for the next bout.' It sounds as if we are discussing a boxing match. He swings his jacket over his shoulder and heads for the door.

'Are you sure you don't want me to see if your wife has any questions?' I ask.

'Nae need. Nowt tae explain!' he says, and disappears around the corner.

On the Monday after Valentine's Day, a GP rang the cancer centre to say that Fergus had a swollen, red right calf. 'Looks like a DVT,' said the doctor. 'Do you have a bed?' Fergus's admission was agreed, and an ambulance was despatched to collect him from home. He arrived within the hour, in a pyjama top and shorts. 'Couldnae get the troosers over ma fat leg.'

Yes, this looks like a DVT: a deep-vein thrombosis, one of the over-clotting complications of cancer. Over the next few hours Fergus has a vein scan to confirm the diagnosis, and begins drugs to thin his blood and prevent the clot from getting any bigger. He tells me about the birthday: about the Boy's joy over his bike, his daredevil pedalling up and down the pavement outside their house on his birthday, and every day since; about Maggie's tears when she saw the locket, and her kissing the photos before hanging it around her neck; about the wonderful dinner she cooked, and the bicycle-wheel birthday cake; about how glad he was to have those special days, without sickness and post-treatment misery. His eyes are shining. Delaying this treatment was the right call, I think, as I leave his room to check my other patients.

The 'cardiac arrest' bleep takes me by surprise. I run to the ward, to find a hubbub outside Fergus's room: a nurse running with the crash trolley, an anaesthetist dashing up the stairs towards us; the patients' tea trolley deserted mid-ward. In Fergus's room he is pale, semi-conscious, panting. His lips are blue. His eyes are wide, surprised-looking. I explain the DVT to the anaesthetist: the likelihood is that the clot in Fergus's leg has broken up and travelled around his veins, and is now blocking the blood supply to his lungs. We give oxygen by face mask: its hissing drowns out the sound of his panting. I ask a nurse to call his wife. The anaesthetist tells me that because of his extensive cancer, and his failing liver, heart and lungs, Fergus is not a candidate for an intensive care unit bed, and I know that this is right – if he is dying, he should do it here, amongst people who know him and with his wife beside him. The crash team withdraws. We wait for Maggie. I give Fergus a small dose of a drug that will take the edge off his breathlessness, and his panting becomes less urgent. I sit beside the bed, wailing inside my head for his loss.

'Am I dying?' he asks me, between deep breaths from his mask.

'You might be,' I answer cautiously, 'but we don't know yet. Maggie is on her way. We're going to stay very close, and if you have any pain I want to know.'

'Bugger!' he says. 'It's too soon tae die. Too much to live fer. My Maggie. Oor Boy . . .' He can only manage one word for each breath he takes.

'Fergus, I can give you some more of that medicine for breathlessness any time you want it. It might make you sleepy, though. Do you want to be awake for Maggie? Or would you rather be asleep, and less breathless?'

Before he can answer, Fergus's breathing changes again: slower, grunting, laboured. His pupils begin to dilate. He is unconscious, unresponsive, unaware, dying. The clot has moved deeper. He is not getting any circulation through his lungs, his brain is not getting any oxygen. Within five minutes, his breathing ceases completely.

Maggie is shown straight into Sister's office when she arrives ten minutes later. Sister takes me in and introduces me. I have heard so much about Maggie, yet never met her. I have to tell her that Fergus is dead. I have to say those words slowly, carefully, so she can understand. I sit beside her and explain about the clot in Fergus's leg moving to his lungs, stopping him from getting oxygen. I explain that we managed his breathlessness so that he was calm and comfortable. I tell her about his joyful recounting of their son's birthday. I repeat his last words, 'My Maggie. Our Boy . . .'

Together, we walk to his room, where the nurses have removed the drips and oxygen pipes and he lies quiet, pale, fragile in his bed. I show Maggie where to sit so she can touch him, hold him, talk to him. I tell her she can sit here as long as she likes.

Later, back in Sister's office, she sips a cup of NHS tea-with-sympathy with Sister while I write out a medical certificate of death for her to take away. I ask if there is anything else she would like to know.

'No,' she says, slowly. 'I only want to say how glad I am that it was you in here today, looking after him, and not that cow that he saw in the clinic last time.'

I am thunderstruck. What can she mean? I ask what happened in the clinic.

'That doctor told him that there was no hope. He might as well miss a week. It wouldn't make any difference. He didn't tell me until we got home. That cow took all his hope away.'

Sister looks at me. I can hear the blood rushing in my head. *Breathe! Breathe! What did I say? How did he hear that?* I cannot imagine how our clinic conversation could have been reconstituted in this way. I remember asking if I should talk to her. I remember him declining. I wonder what he thought he heard me say.

'That was me, Maggie,' I say. 'I saw Fergus every time he came. I remember seeing him before the birthday.' I recount, as best I can, the conversation we had, the decision to avoid treatment-related misery over Valentine's Day, Fergus's hopes for making happy birthday memories for their son. I watch as she tries to reconcile the image she has of the cow in the clinic with the woman before her, who has talked her through the death of her husband. I can see the struggle to comprehend in her eyes.

'I am so very sorry, Maggie,' I say. 'I don't know what to say to you. Maybe I said it wrong. Maybe he heard it differently from how I intended.'

'Actually,' she says after a long silence, 'I think he said what you just said to me. But I knew that if it was really working well, you wouldn't have given him a week off. He was always hopeful, and I was always expecting disaster. He did have a lovely time. I saw it, he was just so happy. You would never think he knew it was his last chance to celebrate our boy's birthday. Our last Valentine's Day. And maybe he didn't. But I did.'

She sips the tea and strokes the locket hanging at her throat. In the silence, I contemplate the horrible harm I have caused. If I had voiced my concerns with Fergus in the clinic, he might have shared that lonely understanding of the approach of death with his wife. If I had only walked around the corner to where she was sitting, she might have had a chance to ask her own questions, to follow her own, hopeless hunch. They might have been able to say the important things that a couple needs to say on the brink of death. Instead, for this lonely woman, there was no goodbye.

And yet, she is prepared to pardon this inexcusable offence. She understands that her husband preferred to say little, and to know even less, and that I allowed that to happen.

'Sorry I called you a cow,' she says.

'It wasn't you, it was the situation,' I reply.

I don't start to cry until she has set off for home, to tell the Boy. There can be no worse conversation for a mother to have.

Slipping Through My Fingers

The emergency department is a sorting-house where very sick people must be helped quickly so that the opportunity to save life is not lost, while the unavoidably dying must also be rapidly identified and supported to make the best of their final moments. Amongst the people coming to the ED who may not leave alive are those still hoping to be made well, those who never previously suspected they were ill, and those who have lived with ill-health and increasing frailty for some time. Only our honesty about the probable outcomes of the treatments we can offer can enable patients and families to make wise choices about when to accept that life is drawing to its close.

Not all dying is neat and well-prepared. Although the final moments of life follow a reasonably consistent pattern of waning consciousness and automatic breathing, the journey to that point may take a less predictable path. Possibly 25 per cent of all deaths are sudden and unexpected, taking place too rapidly to allow time for any treatment. Yet even in such deaths there is often a known underlying condition, such as heart disease, or simply extreme age, that may make the timing of death unpredictable but that nevertheless foreshadows its approach.

So, if most deaths are at the end of a period of escalating ill-health, and if even the majority of sudden deaths are as a result of acknowledged significant illness, why are we still so often unready?

Kathleen, one of our nurse specialists, and I were making our recommendations to staff about a patient well known to the city's palliative care services, who had been brought to the emergency department by her anxious daughter, when a familiar, pink-faced junior doctor ran past us shouting, 'Cardiac arrest Bay 2! I think we'll need you, Pallies!'

When I qualified as a doctor, the specialty of palliative medicine had not yet been established, and palliative care was a concept confined to a few charitably funded hospices. Now I am a consultant in the discipline, and trainee doctors come on placements in our hospital palliative care team. How times have changed. Each year we take three newly qualified doctors for a four-month placement.

Eighteen months ago Lisl arrived in our office, timid and daunted by the idea of working in palliative care. Four months later she had learned new communication skills, could offer a comprehensive pain and symptom assessment, had begun to elaborate her own script for the 'explaining what dying is like' conversations, and had taken to referring to our team members as the Pallies. We love watching each trainee grow in confidence and understanding, becoming ready to take a better understanding of palliative care back out into the rest of their medical practice. Lisl was now a trainee in trauma surgery; palliative care skills are useful in all medical disciplines.

We took up Lisl's invitation, joining the dashing crash team along the corridor to Bay 2. An elderly man had been brought in by an ambulance crew. His heart had stopped in the ambulance, and resuscitation was commenced. Two ED nurses had taken over the resuscitation effort, and Lisl joined them as an anaesthetist prepared to place a breathing tube into the patient's throat. The paramedics were briefing the ED team, and we joined them. Across the room I noticed a middle-aged man in shirt and tie standing horror-struck and white-faced as he watched the scene unfold. A relative of the patient?

I observe as my erstwhile trainee asks the frightened man if his dad had ever discussed resuscitation status. I see him shake his head in disbelief while the resuscitation effort continues like a TV drama. She inserts a second IV line and takes blood for analysis from the patient, while asking his son more questions to fill in gaps in the paramedics' briefing.

It emerges that the patient is eighty-two, with known heart disease and two previous heart attacks, on treatment for high blood pressure and usually limited to walking short distances on the level before chest pain stops him – a classic history of advanced heart disease. Today he developed slurred speech and a weak left arm, then collapsed. His wife called an ambulance, and one of his sons accompanied him to the hospital – the man now leaning against the wall to hold himself up. His brothers and their mother are following by car. My heart sinks – *They'll spend a long time searching for a parking space. They may arrive too late.*

Then the resuscitation team step back. There is a trace on the screen showing that the patient's heart has restarted, but his blood pressure is very low, and there is little sign that his heart is beating effectively. Drugs to support his failing heart are running through an IV line. He is breathing without medical help; an oxygen mask is strapped to his face. The story suggests a stroke, and maybe another heart attack. His chances of surviving are slim; of surviving to become well, remote. There are hard decisions to be made.

Lisl's consultant arrives. He is in charge of ED today. She summarises the man's story, showing him the charts of pulse, blood pressure, oxygen levels, drugs and fluids administered. He nods as she offers her conclusion that this is advanced heart disease, with known poor heart function before today's events; the patient will not benefit from intensive treatment, and he is not a candidate for a heart transplant. The story and some of the physical signs also suggest that he had a stroke this morning, either before or as a result of a further heart attack. This makes it very risky to follow the usual heart attack protocol of using drugs to 'thin' the blood and reduce any clots, because that could worsen a stroke, potentially fatally. The consultant agrees that this situation requires best supportive care until time and events show whether or not there is any potential for the elderly man to recover. He asks Lisl if she is happy to explain the situation to the family, and she nods, moving her hand to indicate the presence of two palliative care staff amongst the busy melee. He smiles at us, says 'Perfect timing!' and departs for his next consultation.

The man in the suit moves cautiously towards his father. He has heard Lisl's words, but as yet I don't know what they meant to him.

The door opens again. Two more middle-aged men and an older lady peer through – the rest of the family has arrived. I don't want to take them away to talk to them in case the man dies while they are not in the room with him. Kathleen realises that there are no chairs for the family and sets off to sort this out. The rest of the team scatter to gather drugs, make phone calls, check on other patients. Only the family, Lisl and I are left with the patient and an ED nurse. I introduce ourselves, and explain that I am a consultant physician in the hospital, that it looks likely that their dad/her husband has had a stroke, and then a period when his heart stopped, and that now his heart is not really beating well enough to support his body. Kathleen materialises silently, carrying chairs; the men sit down, but their mother remains standing resolutely beside her husband, and I am touched to see the young doctor join her, taking her hand to place it in her husband's, which lies motionless on his chest, and then place her own soft hand over them both, nodding at the woman to show that this is allowed – this is her space and time with her husband.

The ED nurse moves quietly between the flashing monitor screen, the drip tubes and the patient, responding to the falling blood pressure, the rapid heart rate, the dropping oxygen levels in his blood; adjusting oxygen flow; changing IV bags; communicating with Lisl using nods and pointing to avoid disturbing our delicate conversation. Kathleen takes a chair amongst the men and watches thoughtfully, face full of compassion.

I ask the men whether they knew their father had a bad heart, and they nod, murmuring that he's been 'a creaking gate' for years. They have been expecting a bad-news phone call any time since his second heart attack two years ago. I ask how their dad has been recently, and they describe a man confined to his home by chest pain and exhaustion. So they realised he was on borrowed time, I comment, and they nod. This is no surprise to them.

'So,' I ask them, 'what did your dad say he would want us doctors to do if his heart got worse, if he collapsed or needed to come into hospital?'

There is a long, tense pause. The men sit, hunched forwards and hands clasped before them, and they look at me with round, frightened eyes. They shake their heads. They don't know what their dad would want.

'Did he ever say anything that would help us to know what to do now?' I ask them, as gently as I can, and one of them replies in a croak of heartbreak, 'He tried to. Oh, God – he tried to talk about it, and I told him not to be so maudlin . . .' His voice cracks and his shoulders heave. Kathleen touches his shoulder gently. A brother picks up the thread. 'Not just you, Sam,' he says. 'Dad asked me to do one of those attorney documents in case Mum ever needed a hand, and I just said he'd be here forever and to stop being gloomy . . .' and his voice peters away.

This conspiracy of silence is so common, and so heartbreaking. The elderly expect death, and many try to talk to others about their hopes and wishes. But often they are rebuffed by the young, who cannot bear, or even contemplate, those thoughts that are the constant companions of the aged or the sick.

Then their mother speaks. She has been gazing at her husband, but listening attentively and making occasional eye contact with me as I spoke to her sons.

'Let him go,' she says quietly. The men sit up and stare, and one begins to object, but she raises her free hand and flaps at him to be quiet. 'He's not living. He's not happy. He often says he's ready to die,' she tells them. She turns to me. 'He knows the lads will look after me, and he knows I'll be all right. He's been ready to die for a long time.' There is utter silence, broken by a sob from one of the men.

'Tell us what he would say if he was awake enough to tell me now,' I encourage her.

She looks down at his face with a fond and familiar smile as she replies. 'He says to me almost every week, "Jeannie, we've had a great life. Now it's time to go. I hope it's soon, and I hope it's sudden, and I hope it's me before you . . ." and I just say, "Gerry, I hope I'm not far behind." And then we have a little cuddle and we feel better.' She pauses, then asks me, 'Will he wake up again, doctor?'

'I think it's unlikely,' I say, awkwardly aware that in the rush of arrival there have been no proper introductions. It seems presumptuous to call her Jeannie.

'Can you see his heart monitor there?' Lisl points out the trace to the family. 'It shows us that Gerry's heart is trying to beat, but it's not strong enough to circulate his blood properly. Without a good blood supply to our brain, we can't be awake. Gerry is unconscious. He is very, very sick . . . He is sick enough to die.' She pauses to let them digest this news.

'Sometimes, even unconscious people are aware of sounds around them, so he may be able to hear your voices and be glad that you're here. We have to decide quickly how intensively to treat him, and we want to do what he would want. We can't ask him, because he is unconscious. That's why we need you, who know him the best, to tell us what he would say. We're not asking you to make the decision – doctors have to make the medical decisions. But if you think there are treatments that he wouldn't want, we will take his views into account as we decide.'

The men swap anxious glances, while their mother looks on. Lisl continues, 'In a few minutes we'll find a bed for him instead of this ambulance stretcher, and a room where you can sit with him. I'm going to make those arrangements now. If time is short for him – and it may be – is there anyone else who should be here?' She waits, and they stare miserably at each other, silent and stunned. 'Why don't you think about that, while I go and find out about a room for him?' I watch her managing an ED death, and admire her confidence and calm compassion – our former trainee, putting her palliative care training into practice.

Nodding at each tearful face, she makes her exit, leaving me to prompt the family, picking up the script where she left off.

'Sometimes, when time might be short, people just want time to be together,' I say. 'Some people have religious beliefs and would like a chaplain or prayers. Some people want music, and some prefer quiet. We want to help you to make this time the best that we can, so please let us know what we can do to help.' *Pause*. This is a lot to take in, and often needs to be repeated. The nurse opens another vial to add to the IV line, and I see that Gerry's blood pressure is almost unrecordable. He is failing fast.

A bed is wheeled bumpily into the room by two nurses, who skilfully transfer him into it, complete with his tangle of tubes and drip lines. They invite the family to accompany them, and wheel Gerry away to a quiet room. Kathleen shepherds the sons, and Lisl takes the wife's hand as they follow. The resuscitation bay is left empty. The ED nurse immediately begins the process of cleaning all surfaces, restocking all drugs and equipment, and preparing for the next potentially life-saving use of the bay. No time for tears.

Kathleen and I leave the ED half an hour later. Gerry is in a single room with his family around him, and the medical team is explaining that he will probably die in the next twenty-four hours of his latest heart attack, now confirmed by blood and heart tests. He is too unstable for a scan to detect whether he has also suffered a stroke, but the answer is academic. His wife has represented Gerry's wish not to have his dying protracted by medical treatment, their sons have accepted their mother's knowledge of the wishes that their dad tried to discuss with them, and the medical team has taken his known preferences into account, deciding not to escalate his treatment to the ICU, where they could certainly prolong his dying but are unlikely to restore his health.

*

I phone Lisl before I leave work that evening, to tell her how well she managed that very difficult conversation. She is pleased to have the feedback. Gerry had died a few hours earlier, and Lisl reported, 'He did that thing that so many people do. That "choose the moment" thing. You know – the family was with him from the time he collapsed, right through ED and into the side room. And then when his sons had gone for food, and his wife went outside for a smoke, he just died. He was only on his own for two minutes.'

This phenomenon occurs with such regularity that we often warn families, especially when the dying process stretches over several days, that it may happen. We don't understand it, but we recognise that sometimes people can only relax into death when they are alone. Are they somehow held by bonds of concern for the watchers? Is it the presence of beloved people in the room that holds them between life and death? Are they choosing? We don't know the answers, but we recognise the pattern.

'Do you ever get used to it?' she asks me. 'Those dying conversations – will I ever just feel OK while I'm doing them?'

The answer, I am glad to say, is no. It will never feel comfortable to sit so close to others' grief. Working in the face of death will always feel profound, numinous and sometimes overwhelming – that's why we work in teams. But you will be able to recognise that you are offering something vital, transformative and even spiritual: the opportunity for individuals to meet or to watch death with an awareness that is lost if we fail to be truthful. The dreadful reality, told with honesty and compassion, allows patients and their families to make choices based on truth, instead of encouraging the misleading, hopeless quest for a medical miracle that promotes futile treatment, protracts dying and disallows goodbyes.

Today, in ED, Lisl's skills focused not on saving life at any cost, but on enabling goodbye. Sometimes, in the end, it's all we have to offer.

Talking About the Unmentionable

One of the many parallel journeys in my life so far has been the journey to young adulthood of my two children, and their introduction to the essential concepts inherent in the human condition – matters as diverse as how the dirty socks from your bedroom floor become clean pairs in the drawer again; why feeding the goldfish the right food in the right amounts is important; where babies come from; why honesty matters; where babies really come from – and this has included their introduction to the concept of mortality as illustrated by goldfish, old people, and eventually by people we love and will miss.

Telling children about death is important, yet uncomfortable. We want to protect them from sadness, but prepare them for life. Children's ability to understand concepts like time, permanence, the persistence of unseen objects, and universality develops over the years, so what we say will be received and processed differently depending on the age of the child. Despite being aware of this in theory, I have been taken by surprise on occasions by the reinterpretation of our conversations by one or other of the children.

Here are some examples from our family journey that show how these early experiences can mature into an understanding of death; and in some cases, how the misunderstandings can be comedic.

Something Fishy

My grandfather died when I was in my thirties and our younger child had recently started nursery. At the time, we had pets: two goldfish, and a cat that had been bequeathed to us by a hospice patient. Great effort went into saving the fish from being lovingly overfed by the children or lovingly consumed by the cat. The idea was that, in observing the life cycle of pets, our children could be gently introduced to matters of fact like not being afraid of water (Check: both are excellent swimmers), looking after things (Check: both are gentle with the fish and cautious with the cat), illness and healthcare (Check: cat-pampering after injections from the vet), and even death eventually (but all three pets were determinedly showing robust good health).

So when I heard that my beloved grandfather had died quite suddenly from a chest infection, I explained to the children, aged three and seven, that I was going to see Grampee now that he was dead, for one last time. I would go and stay with Nana and Grandad, who are very sad, and they would come a few days later with Daddy for Grampee's funeral. As I prepared to set off the next morning, I noticed that one of the goldfish (the spotty one called Ladybird) was swimming strangely, at an odd angle, and moving its gills and fins only on one side. *Can goldfish have strokes?* This fish was definitely looking peaky, but I had an early train to catch, and the family was sleeping. This might be a situation to leave to Super-dad.

That evening, after I had been to the chapel of rest with my parents, and kissed the cold forehead of that strangely unfamiliar face, I was phoned by the children. 'Mummy, Ladybird died,' my three-year-old daughter solemnly informed me. 'But don't worry, we put her in a jug in the fridge so that you can see her.'

The children were not very interested in the funeral, but enjoyed the reunion with their cousins afterwards. The dead fish was a huge topic of discussion, my pair displaying their new expertise to their cousins. My sisters were alarmed to hear that the kitchen fridge was being used as a mortuary, but Super-dad is a pathologist – that's the way he rolls.

I was reunited with Ladybird about four days after her death. She was lying in state in my measuring jug, looking slightly green at the gills. I held her on a tissue on my palm and talked to the children about death. 'Look,' I said. 'She isn't moving; not even breathing. She doesn't feel anything, hear anything, know anything. She isn't sad or afraid. She has no pain. She doesn't even know she's dead.' They stared and nodded. One of them prodded her gently with a clothes peg, as though checking.

'When animals and plants die, their bodies gradually turn back into soil,' I explained, 'and that helps new plants to grow, and makes new food for other animals.' Warming to my theme, I asked them to choose a place in the garden where we could bury Ladybird, so her body could turn into soil and help our plants to grow. They helped me dig a hole under a shrub, and we buried the fish in its Kleenex shroud.

A few weeks later, a visiting friend noticed we were one fish short, and asked what had happened. Our daughter fixed her with big, serious eyes and used her 'explaining voice' to say, 'Ladybird got sick, so Mummy put her into a hole.' *Still a bit of work to do there, it seems.*

Before the age of around five, children do not understand the irreversibility of death, nor that death renders the body totally non-functional. Although my seven-year-old was content to bury a permanently dead and non-functional fish, his three-year-old sister was quite perplexed about the whole situation. And probably a bit anxious about becoming unwell herself!

Plaques

At eight, number-one son was obsessed by the idea of death. It was a phase, but it was driving me crazy, making it hard to separate life from work. Take memorial plaques on public benches, for instance. He was convinced that these marked places of death, as though members of the public risked annihilation each time they sat on a park bench or unwrapped their packed lunches on a seat by the riverside. 'Did they die here, on this bench?' No, the bench was put here after they died. 'So did they die here on the road/falling over that cliff/in this park?' No, this is a place where their family like people to remember them. After weeks of interrogation about bench plaques, which pop up everywhere once you are trying to avoid them, he finally got it. Phew.

One weekend we were out walking in the wilderness. High on the crags was a bench with a plaque commemorating a dad who had died on this very spot, while out mountain-biking with his son. 'Coo-ool,' murmured number-one son reverently. 'Dad, can we bring our bikes here?'

Weeks of work undone in an instant, and the craze began again . . .

This apparently morbid fascination with death is a normal phase of child development. As well as plaque-curiosity, for our son the phase included drawing funerals and coffins associated with long stories about the people in his pictures. This all helped him to place death in a context of, for example, applying to old people, or being the outcome of illness or accidents.

Some time around the age of seven, children become aware that death happens to everybody, and a little later, that it will even happen to them. This may lead to a period of anxiety and frequent requests for reassurance that immediate family members will not die. We addressed this during their childhood by explaining to our children that mummies and daddies don't usually die until they are old and their children are grown-up. Of course, not every family has that good fortune, and specialist advice is available for families helping children to deal with death – see the Resources section at the end of this book for more information.

Cat-astrophe

We moved house to live in the country, our little family, when our daughter was nearly six and her brother nearly ten. The apparently immortal hospice bequest cat was at least sixteen, and the surviving goldfish still outwitting him. It was a big decision, and a good move. There was a huge garden. We grew vegetables and dug a pond, we had access to a river for damming/paddling/fishing in, we released the goldfish into the pond and gave him lots of stickleback friends who were so happy that they multiplied greatly. The cat and a local heron hunted at the margin.

The cat, in particular, thrived. It turned out that he was a skilful hunter, and he would forage far afield, returning with gifts of field mice, bank voles, occasional birds – he once even dragged a rabbit through his cat-flap. These he laid out for display in the garage, a habit the children gradually learned to forgive and eventually even to admire. So by the ages of eight and twelve, they were unusually familiar with the state of *rigor mortis* in these feline trophies.

Although our house backed onto fields, it sat on a busy road, and this was to prove our hunter's downfall. One day, after work, I was drawn to the front of the house by tooting car horns and saw the cat sitting in the middle of the road, surrounded by fast-moving traffic. As I walked out to him, raising a hand to stop the cars, I realised that his back was twisted and his hind legs and tail were not moving – he must have been run over.

Our childminder was about to go home, but she took one look at the cat and then at my eight-year-old daughter and said, 'I'll stay here. You take the cat to the vet.' We quickly found a strong cardboard box (no need to restrain the cat in his animal carrier) and lined it with a blanket. Then my son, twelve going on fifty, climbed into the back seat of the car with the cat in his box beside him, and we set off. I could see both passengers in my rear-view mirror. The cat was panting with his tongue hanging out, glassy-eyed. Every now and then he mewed weakly.

'Why don't you talk to Oskar?' I said to my son. 'Just let him hear your voice. You could touch his head very gently, too. He likes his ears tickled, doesn't he? Just don't touch his back in case it hurts him.'

And so we hurtled the fifteen miles to town and the vet, with my son murmuring encouragement to the cat. 'You're a great cat, Oskar. You're OK. We're here. I'm by you, don't worry. We'll look after you. You're such a great cat.'

I was able to observe changes in the cat's apparent consciousness; he seemed to drift off, and would then suddenly mew and waken again. I realised that this is a pattern I see every day at work – the cat might die during the journey, and my son was unprepared.

'Can you see how comfortable he gets as you talk to him?' I said. 'He's drifting off, isn't he? And can you hear how his breathing is changing too? It's gentler now, isn't it, and slower than it was before? That tells us that he's very comfortable and relaxed, but also very poorly. He must be so glad that you're there to talk to him.'

The boy's eyes fill with tears, his voice wobbles, but he carries on his litany of praise. 'You are the best hunter. You catch all those mice, and you love to chase the birds, and even the rabbits. You are so brave. You are such a great cat, Osk.' And then, 'Stay with us, Oskar. Don't die. The vet will help you. We're nearly there . . .'

The childminder has phoned the vet. They are expecting us, and after one glance at the cat's back they tell me to take him to the animal hospital nearby. They will call and let them know. We get back in the car and drive, very gently now, down the winding road towards the hospital. But the script has changed. From the back seat I hear, 'You're the best cat, Oskar, and I love you. Thank you for being my cat. You have been such a great cat, Osk. We all love you. We could never have had a better cat than you, Osk . . .' *Such a slight change, but that is the past tense. The boy knows that this is goodbye.*

Oskar survived to reach the animal hospital, but died later that day. We brought him home. He is helping the plants to grow in our garden, on his hunting grounds.

Arrival at Destination

My godmother, my mum's sister, is dying. She has developed a brain tumour in her eighties. She is having difficulty finding the right words, but understands everything that is said to her. She has declined radiotherapy ('It will only add feathers,' in her opinion, which translates to mean longer life without quality if her mind is impaired), and accepts that her life expectancy is short. She is worried about who will look after her semi-invalid husband ('I am the fat as a diddle one here!'), but is otherwise at peace.

She managed her birthday at home with a lot of support from family and neighbours, but has had a series of seizures and has been admitted to the huge, indescribably ugly hospital in her city. She is on a medical ward in a side room, and the blinds rattle in the draught from the badly sealed windows. The warmth of the staff, though, makes up for what their building lacks. The hospital palliative care team has been in, and the ward team has been told to expect 'my nephew, she's a proper specialist in all this stuff'. Despite this mixed-gender advertisement of my expertise, they are welcoming and kind. 'Your auntie's lovely,' they tell me, 'and she's dead proud of you!' Then they realise that the D-word has been used, and withdraw, pink-cheeked.

I have travelled by train to the hospital with my daughter, now seventeen. My parents are on their way by car, and my son has picked us up at the station because this is his university town. It's a long time since we buried that fish (and also eventually the cat, several hamsters, the other fish, and the rabbits that were decapitated by our local fox), and he is now a tall, muscular rugby forward, a master of revels, his voice still loud with the joy of living. His sister is gentle and quiet, more reserved, more inclined to ponder first and speak later, to intuit others' feelings and to quietly take a lonely hand in hers.

We enter Auntie's room. She is tiny and pale in a big hospital bed. She is wearing a hospital gown, and the yellow trim jars with her complexion. One of my cousins is in a chair beside the window. He looks up with a face of desperation; he doesn't know how to be, yet he has travelled half a day to sit here, to be available, to show his love. Auntie seems to be sleeping, but my gentle giant booms, 'Hello, Auntie! I like your fancy pyjamas!' and she opens one eye and smiles, recognising the people in the room one by one, beams to see us all, then fills up with tears, declares, 'You've all come such a long day!' and starts to cry. My parents arrive and greet the grandchildren, the nephew from afar, and then Auntie, whom they have been visiting daily. Her face droops on the right and she cannot move her right arm. I notice that my cousin is sitting on the right-hand side of her bed – she has probably not been able to see him. The brain tumour is slowly removing her ability to see, feel, notice, move or interact with the right-hand side both of her body and of her world.

We all find chairs and sit down. I bring my cousin around to Auntie's left, and she is delighted to see him. I have a tube of hand cream in my pocket; I take Auntie's clawed right hand and ask my daughter to take her left hand, and together we massage the cream into her skin. She smiles and says, 'That has a nice taste.' Sporadic sickroom conversation spills around the room. My parents look tired. My daughter is being brave, but sees the grief in her relatives' faces. 'Come on,' I say to my offspring, 'let's see if we can find a cup of tea for everyone.' We take to the concrete corridors, following signs for the café. The gentle giant leads the way (he is a regular in A&E here, through his frequent rugby accidents) while his sister and I follow. She is pale, quiet and tense.

'I am so proud of you two,' I say as we search for the café. 'You're doing everything so well. You've made conversation, you've been kind to your grandparents, you've been so gentle and loving to Auntie.'

'Well, Mum,' says the gentle giant, 'you and Dad have spent a lifetime preparing us for this. No one else at school ever talked about death. It was just a Thing in our house. And now look – it's

OK. We know what to expect. We don't feel frightened. We can do it. This is what you wanted for us, not to be afraid.'

We reach the café. I hug them both. I am not sure that my Big Man speaks for both of them: my gorgeous girl looks tearful and anxious. But that is normal too. Because we *can* do this. We can walk with Auntie for the last few days of her life, loving her and measuring her important contribution to our lives, knowing what to expect as she sleeps more and wakes less, knowing that she will become less able to talk, knowing that the end will be gentle.

And when it comes, in fact several weeks later, it is gentle. She is ready. And so are we.

By being open and honest, we hope that we have made it safe for our children to ask their questions, voice their anxieties, and recognise their sadness at the finality of death. It hasn't made them maudlin; it hasn't made them afraid of taking risks and seizing life's opportunities; they seem to have survived our efforts intact.

Every family will find its own way to deal with the Facts of Life; we need to remember that the Facts of Death are just as important to acknowledge and discuss.

The Sound of Silence

It can be daunting for a family to discuss bad news. Sometimes, if the bad news is broken only to the patient, or only to a family member, that individual can find themself with the burden of knowing a truth they dare not speak. This can lead to a whole conspiracy of silence that isolates people from each other at the very time they need to draw upon each other's strength and support. It is possible to be lonely despite being surrounded by a loving family, as each person guards their secret knowledge for the love and protection of another.

When clinicians break bad news, they would do well to ensure that the right people are present to hear it, to reflect upon it and to support each other in dealing with it. This allows families to share their sadness or worry, and avoids locking anyone away in the Cage of Lonely Secrets. Such difficult conversations can be a challenge in a busy clinic or on a ward round, yet not to do so is a great disservice to the patient and their extended support network – as I had previously found out in an unforgettably shocking way.

It's a bright spring morning. I am knocking on the front door of a terraced house in a coalmining community where the mine closed decades ago and the young people now head for the city at the first opportunity. The older generations, parents and grand-parents, are still a tight-knit community, and the local GP has asked for advice on managing the abdominal symptoms of a woman with advanced ovarian cancer now beyond rescue by the available treatments. She lives with her husband of fifty years in the house they moved into when he was a proud miner and she was his perfect bride.

I wait on the doorstep, and watch a butterfly flit through the minute but beautifully kept front garden. A lawn the size of a large paving stone is surrounded by mature shrubs with swelling flower buds, and bluebells, white narcissi and the brave points of tulip bulbs head for daylight beneath them. The fading daffodils have been deadheaded and their leaves tied into curled knots. This is the work of a fastidious gardener.

Through the frosted glass I see a figure approaching the front door, which cracks open to reveal an anxious face with a finger on his lips.

'Are you from the hospice?' he asks nervously, without opening the door enough to admit me. When I begin to say yes, he shushes me, vibrating his forefinger against his lips, and says, 'She doesn't know! Come in quietly.' Opening the door wide, he ushers me into a tiny, tidy front parlour overlooking the lovely garden. There are ornaments and knick-knacks in wondrous abundance: china figurines, exotic seashells, clay models made by children, porcelain animals, and an assortment of model miners and mining equipment carved from coal. The collection flows across a sideboard, fills a tall corner cabinet, garnishes a Victorian mantelshelf and cascades along the curved bay of the window ledge, all spotless and shining, obviously polished and dusted with obsessive regularity. Apart from us, there is no one in the room. *Where is my patient?*

The man gestures me to sit down. He remains standing, shifting anxiously from foot to foot as he says, 'You mustn't tell her. She couldn't cope with bad news. Trust me, I know her.'

'Tell her what?' I don't know whether he means don't mention hospices, or don't mention her diagnosis.

'She doesn't know it's cancer. She thinks it's just fluid in her tummy, and that the doctors are looking for a treatment,' he whispers urgently, glancing sideways to check that he has closed the door. 'It would kill her if she knew the truth.'

Oh dear. This is awkward. He does know her best, yet when families try to 'protect' a beloved person, it almost always backfires. I have seen it many times. I know I am his guest, and in his house I must respect the house rules. I also know that he is not my patient, and that I am here to do the best I can for his wife. I will have to tread a careful, respectful and kind line, to ascertain what is best for her without frightening him so much that he asks me to leave or diverts the conversation.

I ask what he would like me to call him. Mr Arthurs? He relaxes a little and says, 'Call me Joe. And she's Nelly. Short for Eleanor.'

'Thanks, Joe. I'm Dr Mannix, but most people call me Kathryn.'

Next, I tell him that I am glad that he has warned me. 'You do know Nelly best, and I know that you're working very hard to look after her and to stop her from worrying. How long have you been married?'

He tells me that they were childhood sweethearts, and that they celebrated fifty years of marriage a few months ago. He points to a china plate mounted on the wall, with a picture of Queen Elizabeth II on it. 'That's our golden wedding present from the family. We're great admirers of the Queen,' he says proudly. 'She keeps very high standards. Some people don't value standards any more.'

'Joe, I'd really like to meet Nelly and see how I can help her. Please come with me, so you can check that I'm saying the right things.' He sits on the arm of a chair, looking less tense. 'I promise I'll only answer the questions she asks me,' I continue, 'but I won't promise to lie to her. If she asks me for the truth, I'll have to tell her as much as I think she can manage. Can you trust me?'

Joe avoids my eye, and rubs imaginary dust off the back of his chair.

'No cancer talk?' he asks.

'Not unless Nelly brings it up herself,' I say, and with this he appears content. He conducts me out of the tidy room and up the narrow stairs to a bedroom above the parlour. Here, amidst floral bedspreads and scatter cushions, propped up on pillows, is Nelly, the light of Joe's life.

'This is a different doctor, Nelly,' he tells her, while looking directly at me to give me the clear message, 'Watch your step!'

Nelly holds out a hand to shake mine, then indicates a chair in the window bay, beside the bed, where I should sit. Joe hovers in the doorway, doing his anxious soft-shoe shuffle again. Nelly instructs him to fetch a stool from the bathroom and sit down, for heaven's sake. He grunts and leaves us to retrieve the stool, while I introduce myself. Joe shoots back in like a rocket to check that I am not saying any forbidden words like 'hospice', 'cancer' or 'dying'. I explain that I am a symptom management specialist, and that Nelly's GP has asked for my advice about her swollen tummy. Joe breathes a silent sigh of relief and stations himself on his stool on Nelly's side of the bed. They gaze towards me across a gulf of flowery counterpane.

Through the window beside me I can see a wonderful vista of the local valley, complete with the gauzy green veil of spring unfurling across the woodland along the river. The old pit-head sticks its head above the trees. Nelly is sitting queen-like amongst her pillows, her wasted frame splinted above a pot belly of enormous size. It must be very uncomfortable. Beside her, Joe is perched on his tall stool like a meerkat on guard duty, watchful eyes latched on my face, hand clasping Nelly's.

'Nelly, you've got a fantastic view from your bed,' I start in a place that won't upset Joe. 'Are you feeling well enough to enjoy it?'

Nelly looks towards the window. 'It's like watching a film about the seasons,' she smiles. 'I've seen those trees creep up the pit-head, and before the trees I could watch for Joe walking home from work up the hill. Every minute it's different – the light, the clouds, the colours. I love watching it. Even when I feel so sick . . .'

'Tell me about the sickness,' I invite her, and Joe's neck tenses.

Nelly describes what I am expecting. Her tummy is so swollen she can hardly eat, yet she still has 'stuff inside' that comes up as vomit, in surprising volumes, a couple of times a day. She has a constant sense of nausea. Her bowels don't seem to be working. Her legs are getting wobbly. 'Joe is very patient,' she says, 'and he helps me to walk to the bathroom if I need the toilet. But it's getting tough. I don't seem to have any energy these days . . .'

'Well, you don't eat anything! What do you expect?' Joe interjects sharply. She looks at him calmly and says, 'It's too much of a struggle, love. I do try. I ate that ice cream this morning.'

'What bothers you most, Nelly?' I ask her. 'The nausea? The being sick? The lack of energy? Or something else?' Joe glares at me across the bed.

Nelly pauses before answering. 'It's a mixture of things, really. It's hard to concentrate on anything when you feel sick . . .' I absolutely agree with this. Pain is unpleasant, but it can be pushed from immediate consciousness by sufficiently distracting diversions. But nausea is an overwhelming, all-pervasive, enervating and soul-sapping experience.

'Mainly it's the weakness that worries me,' she continues, 'because it seems to be getting worse. And Joe wants me to eat, and he works so hard to make me lovely snacks, and I hate to see him so sad and disappointed when I just can't face them . . .' She looks at him sadly, and squeezes his hand. 'The worst part is letting Joe down.'

Joe leans forward to protest, but she holds up her other hand for silence, then says, 'Joe, did you offer the doctor a cup of tea?' He shakes his head, and she demands that he do so immediately, where are his manners? A reluctant Joe departs the room, pointing a finger at me and then moving it to his lips out of Nelly's sight. I smile at him, reassuringly I hope, and we hear him lumbering down the stairs.

'What's your main worry about Joe, Nelly?' I ask once the coast is clear. I am not at all surprised by her answer.

'He's just not ready to admit how bad things are,' she says. 'And I can't imagine how he'll manage without me.'

'Without you . . .?'

She looks at me sharply and says, 'You must know it's cancer. They told me months ago, at the hospital. But Joe doesn't know, and I don't know how to tell him. He's a big, brave miner on the outside, but inside he's a soft lad who can't bear anyone to be sad.'

From downstairs we hear a whistle as the kettle comes to the boil. I guess we have a couple of minutes before Joe gets back.

'Do you usually manage big problems all on your own, Nelly? Or in the past, have you and Joe shared things?' I won't try to challenge a preferred way of life for this couple, but I have a sense that they are usually a partnership.

'Ah, we're a great team. Brought up five children together' – her eyes flick to the pit-head beyond the window – 'and weathered many a storm. He may be a softie, but together we're ready for anything.'

'Except this, Nelly?' I ask as gently as I can.

She drops her gaze to her tummy, then fishes in her sleeve and produces a tissue. She wipes her eyes and says, 'It will break his heart. I know I need to tell him. But I don't know how.'

A clinking of china on the stairs heralds Joe's reappearance. He places the tray on the bathroom stool, looks at Nelly, sees her tears and flushes red with fury as he turns to me and demands, 'Are you upsetting my wife?'

'No, Joe, she's not,' interrupts Nelly, firmly yet tenderly. 'Now pour the tea, there's a love.'

Joe turns away to pour, and I can see his hands trembling as he picks up the delicate china milk jug. He glances towards me, checking. I try a smile and tell him I like a big slosh of milk, if he can spare it. He carries on with his task, pouring weak tea for me, medium for himself, and stirring the pot to get a strong mash for Nelly.

'Biscuits, Joe?' Nelly prompts him. 'There should be shortbread in the tin.'

'But . . .' Joe doesn't want to leave us alone again, but she raises an imperious eyebrow and he leaves the room.

'Put them on a nice plate!' she commands as he exits. As soon as she can hear his feet going downstairs, Nelly leans forward over her beachball tummy and says, 'What can I do? How do I tell him?'

It is heart-wrenching to realise how each member of this loving, tender-hearted couple is living a lonely lie in an attempt to save their beloved from distress. The deliberate silence between them is growing as surely as Nelly's cancer, and they may never have a chance to say goodbye unless the deadlock is broken.

'Nelly, what's the worst thing you have ever had to deal with together?' I ask her.

She answers immediately, yet with slow reflection, as though unwilling to hear her own words. 'When our son was killed down the pit. He was seventeen . . . just seventeen. There was an explosion. Three dead. Broke Joe's heart . . . and mine. We only got through by talking. Talking and talking. Saying his name . . . Kevin. No one uses his name any more . . .'

Joe has appeared in the doorway, unnoticed by us as I lean over the bed to catch her softly spoken memories. He sits on the bed, his back to me, and reaches for her hand.

'What's brought this on, pet?' he asks gently, his other hand cupping her cheek and wiping away a tear. She shakes her head sadly and looks down at the bed.

'Joe, Nelly is telling me about your wonderful marriage, and what great partners you are. That you are a wonderful husband, and that together you are a great team.' Joe turns to look at me. Nelly's eyes are fixed on his profile. 'Nelly was telling me that the only way you both got through the heartbreak of Kevin's death was by talking to each other. Over and over.'

Joe looks back to Nelly, who holds his gaze as I say, 'And Nelly thinks she needs to share the tough parts of this illness with you in the same way, don't you, Nelly?'

Nelly nods, gaze locked onto Joe's.

'Nelly, Joe, I've learned so much about you in such a short time,' I continue. My mouth feels dry, my tongue is clicking as I speak. There is so much at stake here, and I want desperately not to make anything worse. 'You love each other so much, and you both want to prevent this illness from making each other sad. You've both told me that.'

Joe draws breath to speak, but Nelly says, 'Listen, love. Just listen.' She is giving me permission to continue.

'Nelly, you told me that you're getting weaker and weaker, and you're worried that you might not get better.' Joe's eyebrows shoot upwards and he blinks at her. 'Joe, you told me that you are so worried about Nelly, but you don't discuss her illness in case you upset her.' It is Nelly's turn to look surprised.

'So it seems to me that, although Nelly is the person who is ill, both of you are suffering' – I emphasise the word slightly – 'suffering from this illness. And each of you is suffering alone. Nelly is upstairs, worrying about Joe. And Joe is downstairs, worrying about Nelly . . . I wonder whether you might bear the suffering better if you could talk about what is going on.'

Nelly gazes at Joe. He moves backwards slightly, as though fearful of what she might say. Nelly, though, is now a woman on a mission. This is her moment.

'I'm dying, Joe,' she tells him simply, and he drops his head and begins to sob. 'I'm dying, and we both know I am.'

'Shush, Nell, no! We can beat this!' he sobs, but she gathers up his hands in hers and says, 'Joe, it's cancer. They told me in the hospital. I just didn't know how to tell you.'

'You knew?' he asks wonderingly. 'You knew all the time?'

'I did, pet,' she says, and he pulls her hands to his lips and weeps.

'I thought I was the only one that knew,' he sobs, 'and I'm watching you fade away. Oh, Nell. My little Nelly.' He is rocking backwards and forwards, crying and kissing her fingers.

Quietly, I rise from my chair and edge around the bed. I collect the tea tray and slip out of the room, picking my steps carefully down the steep stairs with their precious china. They don't need me in there. I will find my way to the tiny kitchen to fill the whistling kettle, and brew up tea-with-sympathy, as I learned to do long ago as an apprentice to Sister of the Gilded China Cups.

Every Breath You Take (I'll be Watching You)

The process of dying is recognisable. There are clear stages, a predictable sequence of events. In the generations of humanity before dying was hijacked into hospitals, the process was common knowledge and had been seen many times by anyone who lived into their thirties or forties. Most communities relied on local wise women to support patient and family during and after a death, much as they did (and still do) during and after a birth. The art of dying has become a forgotten wisdom, but every deathbed is an opportunity to restore that wisdom to those who will live, to benefit from it as they face other deaths in the future, including their own.

'Can you come now?' asks the staff nurse on a ward we know well, sounding somewhat desperate. They are an excellent ward team, and the palliative care team always enjoys working alongside them. She has rung our office because she is concerned that a war is about to break out around the bed of a very poorly patient. The patient, Patricia, has been dying of heart failure for several weeks – initially awake but unable to move far from her bed because of breathlessness and heavy, swollen legs; later, cheerfully bedbound and receiving visitors weighed down with chocolate and fruit (both forbidden by her heart-and-kidney-failure diet, which she simply ignores). Latterly, sleeping for much of the day: the usual pattern, which has been explained to her huge and loving family, who have repeated it frequently to each other like a mantra, as though to calibrate progress as the matriarch approaches death. She has been attended by three daughters, two sons, a bevy of teenage grandchildren – but everyone has been wondering when 'Our Billy' will visit.

Today 'Our Billy' has arrived. Yesterday the ward consultant discussed his mother's status with the governor of the high-security prison where Our Billy is currently detained at Her Majesty's pleasure. The governor agreed that Billy could visit his mother, whose life expectancy would appear to be only days at most. Billy has arrived with his wrists chained to two warders. This suggests that he might wander off, or do harm, if unattended and unshackled. I have found it best not to know the reason for the detention of prisoners, whether patient or family; it is simpler to meet as human being to human being at this already difficult time.

It seems that Our Billy is not happy with his mother's care. Not at all happy. He wants to know when she will wake up; he wants to know why she has been given 'a slug of something' to make her so sleepy; he wants to know when did British hospitals start treating old women worse than animals. Not happy. This ward team is more than capable of dealing with unhappy relatives, even those in chains attached to guards. There must be another dimension to this problem. Sonia, our hospital palliative care lead nurse, heads up to the ward to investigate.

She finds a ward in turmoil. All the nurses are upset. One of the junior doctors is weeping in the doctors' office. The cleaners have just informed Sister that they will only work in Patricia's room in pairs. Sister invites Sonia into her office and closes the door. She explains that 'Our Billy' is the youngest of Patricia's six children, and has always been regarded as her favourite. His sisters describe him as 'spoilt rotten', and his first prison sentence, for – 'Don't tell me, it's better not to know,' Sonia interrupts – so Sister continues her story by saying that Billy has been in trouble with the law all his adult life. His current sentence is in a high-security prison, implying a firearms offence or grievous bodily harm, at least. His sisters are furious with him, and Patricia is now too close to death to realise that Billy is here, for which he blames them, saying they left it too late, they have had Mum sedated, they just wanted to get their own back.

Billy's angry and unpleasant comments have upset the cleaners, he has made personal threats against the nurses, and he has told the young doctor that she is 'rubbish'. The distressed daughters have asked the doctor to give Patricia something 'to wake Mum up so she knows Our Billy is here'. This is not a response to his bullying, but born of their love for their mother, who has missed Our Billy so much. But Patricia is not under sedation, she is simply dying. There is no sedative to reverse. It is the daughters' compassion for their mother and brother, and not Billy's arrogant swaggering, that has reduced the doctor to tears.

Sonia and Sister enter Patricia's room. She is lying on her side, her back to the door, with the head of the bed tilted upright to reduce the waterlogging of her lungs caused by her heart's failure to push blood around her system with any efficiency. She is breathing deeply and slowly, and there is a rattling, bubbling sound with each in-breath and out-breath. Her lips are dusky. Sister introduces Sonia to Carly, the daughter on current Mum-watch, and to Billy, who is sitting between his warders. Sonia greets them all, then moves to the bed and walks around it to Patricia's head.

'Hello, Patricia, I'm Sonia,' she announces, close to Patricia's ear. 'I'm here with Carly and Billy. Can you open your eyes?'

'You daft woman,' sneers Billy. 'Don't you know sedated to death when you see it?'

Sonia ignores him. She watches Patricia's breathing, and measures her pulse. Her breathing is becoming faster and more shallow, but is still bubbling and rattling.

Sonia turns to Carly, Billy and the warders. To everyone's surprise, she addresses the warders first.

'Do you have to use wrist restraints?' she asks them. 'How's the man supposed to cuddle his mum with those on? Does he look like a man in a hurry to leave?' Billy looks startled, and then grudgingly impressed. The warders have a discussion, and decide that the handcuffs and chain can be removed. Billy rubs his wrists in wonder, then stands up. Both warders leap to their feet, but Billy walks slowly towards his mum. He is crying.

Sonia asks the warders to take a seat outside the room. There is only one exit, Billy is safe in here, and he needs some privacy. 'I am the nurse in charge, and I know that I can request this.' Sonia can be magnificent when required, and this is just such an occasion. The ward sister agrees, and Carly gives Billy a thumbs-up sign. The warders leave the room, and Sonia thanks them with genuine warmth as they depart, assuring them that she will take personal responsibility for Billy while he is in the room. She looks at him and says, 'Don't you make me regret this, Billy.' Billy is speechless.

The two senior nurses now turn their attention to their patient. They decide to move Patricia's position in bed, to see if that will reduce the bubbling noise in her breath. With gentle, expert hands they roll her onto her back, ease her upright, adjust and plump her pillows, and slowly lower her down again. They describe aloud what they are doing, talking to Patricia throughout the procedure. Still deeply unconscious, but semi-sitting in bed and supported by pillows under each arm, she is now breathing with slow, gulping breaths, but there is less bubbling.

Sonia rearranges the chairs so that Carly and Billy are sitting on either side of Patricia, each able to hold a hand. Billy tries to lace his fingers between his mum's while Carly strokes her arm.

Sister departs, and Sonia speaks to the family. 'Can you hear how the pattern of her breathing is changing between fast and panting, then slow and snorey?' Billy and Carly look at Patricia, then Carly says that this has been the pattern for a couple of days.

'It's a sign of being deeply unconscious,' says Sonia. 'It means your mum is in a coma. Do you know what I mean?'

Billy tugs at Patricia's fingers. He bites his lip and nods. 'Like a head injury?' he asks.

'Exactly the same process, Billy, but this isn't because of an injury, it's what happens to us all as our brain shuts down. As we're reaching the end of our life.'

She pauses. The room is silent apart from the grunting of Patricia's breathing. No more bubbling.

'We know from people with head injuries who get better,' says Sonia, treading carefully, 'that even deeply unconscious people are aware of the sounds around them. They hear our voices – your voices. Hearing the right voice can make an agitated person calm; hearing a voice they don't like can make people more agitated. That's why the nurses talk to your mum when they're caring for her. We know she's deeply unconscious, but we want to treat her with respect and dignity just the same.'

Billy looks thoughtful. Then he takes a deep breath, and howls, 'Mam, it's me, Billy! I'm here, Mam! I'm here . . . I love you, Mam! I do love you. I'm so sorry . . .' His sobbing prevents him from continuing.

'That's it, Billy, that's exactly the right thing to do. Just keep talking. Talk to her. Talk to each other. Just let her hear your voices.'

Next, Sonia turns her attention to the implications of Patricia's breathing pattern. This is 'periodic breathing', and is a sign that the end of life is approaching.

'Carly, where is the rest of the family?' Sonia asks, and Carly explains that because their mum has been so ill for so long, they have been running a rota to make sure someone is always with her, but that everybody gets enough rest too. Sonia says that this is a wise plan, and it's good to be working with a family that is caring for one another so well.

'But I think the time is coming to get everyone together, Carly, because . . . Listen. Do you hear the long pauses your mum is taking in her breathing from time to time?'

Everyone listens: there is no sound of breathing from Patricia for five seconds, ten seconds, nearly twenty seconds . . . Sonia is on the brink of deciding that Patricia has died, when with a deep, shuddering breath the fast, shallow panting starts all over again.

'This will be the breathing pattern now,' Sonia explains. 'Fast at first, then slower and slower, then a long pause, and then the pattern starts again.' Carly and Billy nod, turning from Patricia to Sonia and then back to their silent mother. 'And one of the times that she's breathing very slowly,' Sonia continues, clear and careful now with this important message, 'she will breathe out, and then just not breathe in again. As gentle as that. And maybe quite soon.' She pauses to be sure they have taken this in, then asks, 'So shall we call the others in?'

Already Sonia can see that Patricia's breathing is gentler. The muscles in her face have relaxed so much that her mouth is open. Time is getting short. Knowing that she is guarantor for Billy, Sonia cannot leave the room, so she presses the nurse call button. Sister pops her head around the door.

'We're just discussing that time may be getting short, Sister,' says Sonia. Her voice is calm, but the nurse-to-nurse communication is clear. 'And Carly should really stay here, so can someone gather the rest of the family?'

Sister understands both the message and the urgency. 'Shall I call Bella first, Carly, and ask her to let everyone know?'

'Yes, tell Bella to tell Gabby, and then just come straight away. I'll text the boys. Tell her I'll do that,' says Carly, flushing and reaching into her handbag for her mobile phone. 'And Sister – tell them Our Billy's here.'

Meanwhile, on a surgical ward in the next block, I am meeting another family around a different deathbed. The patient is Brendan, a middle-aged man who has widely spread cancer of the oesophagus. He is a self-employed carpenter, and although he has had escalating heartburn and a feeling of difficulty with swallowing for months, he has been too busy with work to see a doctor. Now the cancer has blown a hole into his chest from his oesophagus, one of his lungs has collapsed, he has gastric juices in his chest cavity, and he is dying. Our team has been working to manage his chest pain and breathlessness, and today he has been awake and comfortable long enough to talk to his wife Maureen and to say prayers with the chaplain, who has been a great support to them.

I have come to the ward to meet Brendan's brother Patrick, who has just arrived from Ireland. Brendan is lying peacefully unconscious in his bed. His breathing is shallow and slow when I arrive and greet Patrick, Brendan (because we always talk to unconscious people) and Maureen.

'I just can't believe it!' Patrick protests, pacing at the bedside. 'I was only just talking to him on the phone a few days ago, and now look at him! It beggars belief! Why aren't you all doing something? He's a young man! You can't just let him die!'

I take a seat beside the bed. Somehow, sitting gives a message of solidarity, of being prepared to be really present, even if only for a while. I watch Patrick pacing, and see Maureen's taut, stressed expression. It was generous of her to send for her emotional brother-in-law at this difficult time.

Maureen is a compassionate soul. She and I have spent the last few days discussing how she is preparing their teenage sons for the death of their father. She has been inspirational: she has broken the terrible news, brought them to visit him, helped them to tell him how much they love him, explained what will happen as he is dying just as I had explained it to her, and given them the choice about whether to be here or not. Today they are in school (she has even told the school, so her boys will have support), but a friend is on standby to bring them in at short notice if necessary. *Time to address Uncle Paddy's distress, before the boys arrive.*

Brendan's breathing changes again. He enters another period of deep, noisy breathing, and the saliva and secretions at the back of his throat rattle and bubble with every breath, in and out. Paddy pauses his pacing to listen, then shouts, 'Would you listen to that, now? Listen to him! Groaning! He's in agony!'

This is a common situation. People who have never seen anyone die, who are not familiar with the process, can misinterpret what they see and hear. Usually this convinces them that their worst fears are coming to pass. Paddy can hear the throaty rattle of breath through fluids, and the deep, stertorous rumble of periodic breathing, and he thinks that his beloved brother is groaning.

'You wouldn't let a dog suffer like this!' he shouts. 'It's disgraceful! Can't you do something? Can't you just put him out of his misery?'

There *is* someone in this room who longs for his personal misery to end, but it's not Brendan. Brendan is so deeply unconscious that he is neither coughing nor swallowing to clear the liquids pooling in the back of his throat. He is completely unaware of them. Meanwhile, Maureen sits quietly beside his bed, stroking his cheek and talking quietly into his ear about happy times, family holidays, their beloved boys, and telling him that they love him, they love him, they will remember him, they will be OK. Paddy's distress, though, is palpable.

I invite him to come and sit beside me in a vacant chair. He obliges reluctantly. I ask him what he thinks is going on, and he tells me that Brendan is struggling to speak, to express his pain. I ask him to listen with me – quietly, so we can really concentrate. The periodic breathing has moved on to a gentle panting phase; the bubbling rattle persists. I ask Paddy how he would feel if he had fluid in the back of his throat like Brendan has. Would he swallow? Cough? Splutter? 'Of course I would. The tickle would be terrible.'

'So look at Brendan,' I say. 'Look closely. He isn't coughing, or gagging, or swallowing, is he?' Paddy acknowledges this. 'Brendan is so completely relaxed, so deeply unconscious, that he just doesn't feel his throat at all. He has saliva in the back of his throat, and yet he isn't trying to clear it away. And that tells me that he is deeply comatose.'

Paddy looks back at Brendan. He watches closely. He is thinking. 'Well, what about that groaning he was doing before?' he asks suspiciously.

'Ah, that noisy breathing . . .' I begin, but Maureen interrupts and tells him, 'That's just deep breathing. It's a normal noise. He sounds like that when he's asleep at home sometimes. Although he won't believe me . . .' She smiles, and strokes Brendan's face again.

Maureen and I have rehearsed how she will explain the process of dying to the boys. She doesn't want them to misunderstand what they might see. We have talked about the breathing changes: the cycle of deep, noisy breaths turning slower and shallower; the pauses; the restart of the cycle. She is watching Brendan follow this predicted course, and she is taking comfort from it.

Maureen and Paddy stare at each other across the bed. Both are watching the same scene, yet where she is drawing comfort, he is perceiving distress.

'Are you sure now, doctor?' he asks me, and I tell him that this is normal dying, comfortable dying, gentle dying. He will see Brendan's breathing change between fast and slow, shallow and deep. He will see it become more gentle. And then, after one of those exhalations, Brendan will simply not breathe in again. It may be so gentle that it's hard to notice it has happened.

Paddy's eyes spill over with tears. 'Can I stay until then?' he asks Maureen.

She reaches across the bed to take his hand, and says, 'I'm counting on it, Paddy. For Brendan. For me. And for the boys.'

I slide out quietly, to join Sonia in the land of handcuffs.

Patricia is now surrounded by daughters and sons, partners and spouses, grandchildren. Despite the number of people in the room, it is quiet as everyone listens to her breathing. Sonia has joined the warders on chairs outside the room to make space. Sister is supplying trays of tea. Peace has broken out within the family. Sonia and I slip back into the room, where gentle conversation has taken over from the silence. Sonia indicates with her eyebrows that I should look at the patient. Patricia is resting back on her pillows. She looks very still and peaceful. Her eyes are closed, her mouth is open, her skin is white and her fingertips are turning purple. She is not breathing. And nobody has noticed.

'Gosh, she looks peaceful,' says Sonia. 'She must be so glad to have you all here. What do you make of her breathing?' They all look. They stare. Those closest to her touch her chest to test for movement. 'She's just stopped breathing, I think,' says Sonia calmly. 'She could hear that you were all here. She knew it was safe to go. You have all done a fantastic job.'

A quiet sobbing emerges from Our Billy. He walks across the room, gets onto the bed beside Patricia, and buries his face in her neck. 'Goodnight, Mam. I love you,' he whispers. Sonia and I leave the room, inform the warders and the ward sister, and walk back to our office. Our work is finished here. Both families are ready, their mourning can start well, with a good understanding of the peaceful deaths they have just accompanied.

'I love our job,' I remark as we stand in the hospital lift with a newborn baby in a cot, proud parents and a midwife escort.

'What do you do?' asks the midwife, searching for our roles on our name badges.

'Much the same as you,' replies Sonia as the doors open and we walk out. We turn and smile at the new family and the midwife, whose shocked mouth describes a perfect O as the lift doors close.

The thing is, Sonia is right. We are the deathwives. And it's a privilege, every time.

Beauty and the Beast

Bereavement is the process that moves us from the immediacy of loss and the associated grief, through a transition period of getting to know the world in a new way, to a state of being able to function well again. It's not about 'getting better' – bereavement is not an illness, and life for the bereaved will never be the same again. But given time and support, the process itself will enable the bereaved to reach a new balance.

For children, whose mainstay of support in grief is their parents, there is a particular challenge in a dying parent supporting their child, knowing that it is their own death that will precipitate the grieving that will change the child's life. Preparation is key: painful and tragic though it is, this is an act of parental love that is bequeathed to the future that they themselves cannot enter.

The referral letter from the gynaecological cancer nurse specialist says the young woman has pain in her legs. It tells me that she has cancer of her cervix, now expanding inside her pelvis. Her kidneys are beginning to struggle to get urine to her bladder through the mass of cancer. I expect a wreck.

The girl who presents herself in tight jeans, high heels, impeccable make-up and long, dark hair sweeping straight down to her waist is, therefore, something of a surprise. She is not just beautiful, she is stunning. I invite her into the clinic room and she walks with graceful elegance. It is only as she lowers herself into the armchair beside the desk, cautiously supporting her weight with a tight grip on its arms and wincing slightly as her hips flex, that there is any evidence of trouble. She recovers her composure quickly, flicks her hair over her shoulder, and inclines her head towards me with a smile that suggests I am invited to speak.

I begin, as always in the clinic, by introducing myself, and asking what she would like me to call her. She seems taken aback to be invited to call me by my first name, and says her name is Veronica, but I should call her Vronny. 'Only my mum calls me Veronica,' she smiles, 'and that usually means I'm in trouble.'

My next clinic procedure with a new patient is to ask how they hope I may be able to help them. Vronny pauses to formulate a response. 'Well, if I could move around a bit more easy' – she uses the local dialect – 'that would be a great start. The cancer nurse said you was good with pain. That's why I said I'd come . . . to this' – pause, swallow – 'place.'

'You mean a hospice?' I ask, and she nods, holding her breath as tears spring to her eyes. 'Was it a bit of a shock to get the appointment letter with the hospice name on?' I ask, knowing that this has surprised other patients in the past. She nods, and I ask what she thinks hospices are for.

'Well, you come out in a box, don't you?'

'I know a lot of people think that,' I say, 'but I'd be very surprised if people well enough to come to my clinic today need boxes to go home in.' She smiles a thin, unenthusiastic smile.

I offer to explain what a hospice in England in the 1990s actually does, telling her I think it will be less worrying than she seems to expect. She agrees with an anxious 'OK . . .'

'You told me you have a cancer nurse, so I know you know about your cancer,' I begin. 'We see people with lots of different illnesses, not only cancer.' She looks up, surprised. 'The patients we see all have symptoms that are troubling them, caused by their illness. And they are usually serious illnesses. Some people who come here are never going to get completely better, some might actually die here while we're trying to manage their symptoms. But more than half the people who come here for a week or two of care will go home and feel loads better, instead of leaving in a box. That's not what people think though, is it?'

She shakes her head. Not what she was expecting. Surprises all round today, it seems.

I continue, 'Our hospice is more like a specialist hospital ward, only instead of specialising in heart trouble or gynae problems, we specialise in symptom control. Physical symptoms like pain or breathing problems or sickness; and emotional problems that come with serious illnesses like worry, sadness, panic; or family problems, like everyone is taking over and the poor patient feels overwhelmed, or how to tell children that a parent is seriously ill.'

At this last statement she looks up quickly, and I realise that I may have touched a raw nerve. Something to talk about later perhaps, or on another day when she is ready.

'So now you know a bit more about what we do, what do you think we may be able to help with? Because I'm completely out of boxes today, so I was intending to try to help you to feel a bit better.'

And now she smiles, a dazzling and open smile, and says, 'Can you help with the pain in my legs?'

'Tell me all about it, then.' I pick up my pen to take notes as she talks, and I ask extra questions to make sure I have fully understood.

Vronny tells me about her pain and about its impact on her. She is thirty-two, and the mother of a seven-year-old daughter and a nine-year-old son. She lives with her partner Danny, who is the father of her daughter and also 'Dad' to her son. He works as a packer in a local mail-order company, where she was a clerk. The family-run business has been generous with time off for her treatment, and irregular hours for Danny so he can support her.

Her mum lives around the corner, and her two sisters are also nearby. 'It's exhausting keeping on top of things,' she says, 'but I need to keep the place clean so they won't worry.' The trouble is that she wants everything to look 'normal' so people won't think she is ill. Normal includes a fastidiously tidy house ('I can't bear to see a speck of fluff on the carpet!') and her unbelievably tight trousers – I really cannot imagine how she pours herself into them, but undoubtedly she looks both gorgeous and stylish.

She describes a pain that begins in her buttocks and shoots down both legs like electric shocks. It is worse when she bends her hips (as when she lowered herself to sit earlier), and it wakes her sometimes when she turns over in bed. She also has some pain in the lower part of her tummy, where the skin feels strangely tough.

I ask her to undress so I can take a look at her legs. She slides behind the modesty curtain, and I hear her puffing and exhaling with the effort of removing the tight trousers. By the time I pull back the curtain she is lying serenely on the examination couch under a blanket. With her permission, I pull back the blanket to examine her. Chest is clear, heart sounds fine, but the skin over her tummy is imprinted by the shape of the seams and zipper of her trousers, showing me that there is fluid trapped in the skin there, now moulded to the contours of her clothes.

And then we inspect her legs together. The skin is shiny and tight, stretched over the fluid that is trapped in her legs by the pressure of tumour squashing the veins in her pelvis. The muscle power in her legs is normal – I test this by asking her to resist my attempts to bend or straighten each joint, which results in much laughter, particularly when I check her reflexes with my little tendon hammer. But the sensation in her legs is not normal. In the areas where she feels the shooting pains the skin is less sensitive, and she cannot discern the difference between a sharp point and a cotton bud when her eyes are closed.

Pulling the blanket back over her, for warmth and modesty, I observe her anxious face as she awaits my verdict.

'There's nothing we weren't expecting, Vronny. Do you want to get dressed again before we talk?'

'Can you do anything to stop my pain?'

'I think we can help. Do you want a hand to get dressed, and then we can discuss a plan to try to make you feel more comfortable.'

'I'll manage, thanks,' she dismisses my offer briskly, and I leave her behind the curtain. While I write up my notes I hear her struggling to get back into those trousers.

Once Vronny has gingerly reperched herself on the armchair, we discuss the pain in more detail. Pain that is felt in areas where the skin sensation is abnormal is usually due to nerve damage. There are specific treatments that work better than the usual painkillers for nerve pain, and I suggest that she tries one of these. I'll make the recommendation to her GP, who will issue the prescription. She agrees to give it a go.

And then I ask about the trousers. I wonder whether the pressure on the nerves in her pelvis might ease if she wore something looser. Somewhere deep inside Vronny, a dam bursts. She looks straight at me, blinking away the tears that are brimming in her eyes, and takes a deep, shuddering breath. She opens her mouth to speak, but instead emits a hollow, howling sob that shakes her whole body. Then she is convulsed by sobbing, wringing her hands and rocking on the chair. Sitting so close that our knees are almost touching, I silently hand her tissue after tissue for what feels like an eternity, until the wave has passed. She blows her nose and looks at me, murmuring, 'Sorry . . .'

'Do you think you'll be able to talk about what just happened?' I ask gently. I know that the thoughts that trouble us most, our deepest fears and darkest dreads, are usually suppressed and buried, to allow us to get on with daily life. It is only when they break the surface that they trigger our emotional responses. Vronny will be more able to identify those dreadful thoughts now, while her distress is still palpable. But it's a big ask, and she may wish to bury it all back in the darkness.

'I dunno,' is her first response, followed by, 'I'd always thought that if I ever started crying about all this, then I'd never be able to stop . . .' She sniffs again, and stares at the crumpled, damp tissue in her hand. Another sob judders its way out, but it is gentler now. She lifts her chin resolutely and says, 'This is who I am. This is how I look. If I can't look like this . . .' she indicates the trousers and her voice wobbles, but she pushes on, 'then I won't feel like me.'

This is a deep idea, but experience tells me that it may not be the whole of the issue. I invite her to consider what not feeling like herself would mean. It's a hard question, and she furrows her brow as she thinks it through.

'I feel as though I might just disappear. Just stop trying. I might just let the house be a tip, and wear fat pants, and not bother any more. If I let one thing change, then I might lose control of everything.' She gulps and takes a deep breath, but she is now so busy thinking about her thoughts that she is no longer awash with emotion. Here is an important truth in action: by being able to sit with the deepest anguish and not shut it down, it is possible to enable people to explore their most distressing thoughts, process them, and even find more helpful ways to deal with them.

'Losing control of everything sounds horrible,' I agree. 'What exactly would that mean for you?' She is now calm and very focused. After a thoughtful pause she says in a whisper, 'Dying.'

'Vronny, can you bear to tell me what's in your mind when you think about dying?' I ask, passing her a fresh tissue as a sign of solidarity. Taking the tissue, she fixes me with troubled eyes, and says, 'There's no one to tell my daughter about periods,' before dissolving into gentle tears that drip onto her lap while she sits as still as a statue. A weeping Madonna.

'I'm deserting them,' she whispers, as though she can hardly bear to hear the words said aloud.

We sit in silence. I never get used to the variety of deeply personal agonies that the idea of dying can trigger. Vronny's children are a little older than my own. I know that the pain I am feeling is partly my own, projecting myself into her predicament and considering the loss of this precious maternal task.

I had anticipated a simple, one-appointment pain consultation in my out-patient clinic. It could have gone that way, if I had not asked about those trousers. But now I understand that Vronny's distress is not really about the physical pain. She is a woman alone, trying to hold the unravelling threads of her very existence together as her disease progresses. There is work for her to do, and doing it well will allow her children to enter their lives without her in a better-prepared way. She sees herself as the guardian of their happiness, and she is. Their bereavement preparation will be her last act of love for them.

'How much of the time do you spend having these terribly sad thoughts?' I ask. She tells me that she is sad almost all day, every day, and that aggressive vacuum-cleaning allows her to act out her rage at the unfairness of dying so young.

'That gives me a great mental picture of you with your vacuum,' I say. 'Do you wear body armour?'

She laughs. 'Yeah, I think I scare the neighbours!'

Her composure has returned. Now I can discuss where we might go next in helping her. Using a series of questions to help her notice how her strongest emotions are associated with thoughts and images in her mind that she finds almost intolerably distressing, I enable her to consider the possibility of having some help to process that distress, and to devise some plans for how she will cope emotionally as her disease progresses. I explain that, as well as this medical clinic, I also run a clinic dedicated to helping people with this kind of distress, using cognitive behaviour therapy.

'It's exactly what we just did,' I say. 'You can learn how to find the really upsetting thoughts, and then deal with them. For example, who told *you* about periods?'

'My mum. It was terrible. She was so embarrassed. I don't want that for Katy.'

'So how would you choose someone who would do it better?'

She considers, and then says, 'Katy loves my sisters. And her best friend's mum is lovely too. Katy likes sleepovers there, and she stayed with them when I was in hospital.'

'So, of those three, who would you choose? And who do you think Katy would choose?'

'I'll think about it . . . Silly, innit? There was such an obvious answer, and I just didn't see it,' she muses. I point out that being really upset can get in the way of thinking clearly – which is exactly what CBT is designed to help with.

Over the next three months, Vronny and I met for an hour's CBT session most weeks. She learned to notice the way, when she was feeling sad or scared or angry, there was always some thought in her mind driving the emotion. She called them her 'pop-ups'. Many of her pop-ups were thoughts about keeping things 'normal', yet she did allow herself to buy a larger pair of jeans, and decided to buy a soft, smart pyjama suit for daytime wear at home. ('Elasticated waist! Like an old lady! At my age!')

In CBT, we looked at the thoughts and behaviours she used to keep her life on the rails, and tested different ways of doing things. We noticed that she rebuffed all offers of help, but was exhausted by her daily cleaning and vacuuming schedule by the time her children came home from school. She tried the 'experiment' of taking up her sister's offer of calling round to help for an hour each morning, and found that she appreciated the companionship, the help with vacuuming the stairs, and that her whole life did not unwind as predicted. They shared memories of their 'sex education' talks with their mum over a particularly hilarious tea break, and Vronny asked her sister to do the honours for Katy 'when the time seems right'.

'We had a little cry then,' she confided to me, 'but it was a good cry.'

Early on in CBT, Vronny identified the need to prepare Katy and her brother Ben for her death. This led to another ferocious bout of weeping, as she faced and described the haunting picture in her mind of her cherished children, alone and distressed in a school playground, with no one to turn to. This image, she admitted, was often in her mind, and was certainly among her thoughts on the day we first met.

'What would help them most?' was my initial question, and

Vronny easily named several strategies that might help, starting with telling their headmistress about what was happening to Vronny, and asking their teachers to be vigilant for any distress at school; explaining to the children that Mummy is still not well, and she might sometimes be too tired to talk much, but she will always love them; and marrying Danny, so he can be named Ben's legal guardian after her death. 'He keeps asking me,' she said, 'but I feel too fat and heavy to be a proper bride.'

The most daunting task Vronny set herself, though, was the preparation of memory materials for Katy and Ben. She had a family photograph collection, contained in three huge biscuit tins, but when she tried to sort through it and choose which photos she would write short notes about, so that Ben and Katy could have her memories of those occasions when she was no longer there to ask about them, she felt overwhelmed.

'So I knew what to do,' she told me in one CBT session. 'Since I come here to think about the upsetting stuff anyway, I decided we could do that here too.' She opened her shopping bag and produced two tins of photographs. 'I've sorted them into a tin for Katy and a tin for Ben, but I want to put them in albums, and write about where we were and what was happening then, and what I can remember – like I would if I was talking to them when they're bigger. Also,' she added shyly, 'I'm not a good speller. I thought you could help with that too.'

My heart sank. I have spent my professional life with people facing death, and I have self-protection strategies to deal with that, but my discomfort zone is bereavement. I avoid bereavement preparation work – I find it simply too heart-rending. But Vronny was not willing to have any other 'sad' sessions, even with a highly skilled children's bereavement specialist. So, with me taking advice (and support) from our bereavement specialist, Vronny and I extended our hour a week to include twenty minutes' 'children time'. It was both intriguing and terrible to hear her describing family memories, and help her to capture those lost happy times on notes, written in her round, childlike hand and attached to each photograph. She wrote letters for their eighteenth and twenty-first birthdays. Together we assembled two time capsules in those biscuit tins, to entrust into her children's uncertain future without her.

'I'm going to marry Danny, by the way,' she dropped in coolly. She was trying to sound casual, but her grin was as wide as the sky.

She was a beautiful bride, of course. Beaming and radiant, resting on Danny's arm, holding Katy's hand and kissing Ben's head in the photograph she chose for both their collections.

As a wedding present, I gave her two big photograph albums, one in a pretty butterfly design and the other decorated in the colours of Ben's favourite football team. She knew what they were for.

I wonder where they are now.

Contemplation of one's own death is a complex affair. Some people fear the approach of dying, others fear the moment of death, a few long to get it over with. Some fear ceasing to exist, others fear continuing to exist in an unimaginable way, and others hope for a promised paradise. Some experience the sadness of anticipated separation from loved ones, and others feel jealous of those who will survive without them. It is simply impossible to guess what another person means when they are considering their mortality. In palliative care, we have learned to make no assumptions: we ask. The interesting thing is that people are able and willing to answer, and when they share that burden they often discover, from within themselves, new insights and ideas that help them to cope.

Pause for Thought: Naming Death

Notice how often you hear euphemisms like 'passed', 'passed away', 'lost', in conversations and in the media. How can we talk about dying, plan our care or support those we love during dying, theirs or ours, if we are not prepared to name death? Do you and your family avoid the D-words? If you do, how could you begin to change this?

If you were approaching your own death, who would be the important people to tell? Who do you hope would tell you if they knew that their death was approaching?

Is death something the younger members of your family feel allowed to talk and ask about? Don't assume because they never mention it that they don't know. Just like Joe and Nelly, even young children may try to avoid upsetting adult family members if they get the idea that a particular subject will cause distress if spoken about.

How do you and the people you are closest to make their views known? Do you all like to tell people clearly, or do some of you prefer to drop hints? How good are the rest of you at picking up each other's cues?

Do you know what kind of care your loved ones would like as their life's end approaches? Or have you assumed that what you would like is also what they would like, or that you will be able to guess if you need to?

If you were close to dying, would you prioritise being as awake and alert as your condition would allow, or would you prefer to be sleepier and less aware of the situation and the people around you?

What balance do you see between the length of time you live, and the quality of life you are living? Do you think that, if you had a choice, you would choose to accept or to forgo treatments that extend your life if they do not restore quality? Would you prefer to live for as long as possible, even if it means being supported by machines in an intensive care unit, or to make plans that declare at what level escalation of treatments should stop, to focus on comfort instead of prolonging life? Do you feel confident that, if you suddenly became life-threateningly ill, your closest family and friends would know your wishes and preferences about your care?

These are big questions. They may take several conversations to work through. Do consider taking the time to discuss them now, rather than waiting until it becomes a matter of life or death. The staff in the emergency department, the rapid response team or the ambulance crew will be glad to know that you have made your wishes clear. And so will the loved ones who are charged with the responsibility of representing your views at a very challenging time.

If you already have a serious medical condition, consider asking your GP or hospital specialist about what particular emergency situations it would be wise to plan for. In many areas, people can have plans written to describe what care to put in place if a foreseeable crisis arises. This avoids emergency ambulance dashes and unnecessary or unwanted hospital admissions, whilst making sure that people whose crisis requires an urgent response (and sometimes appropriate admission to hospital) get what they need. You can also request clarification of whether or not a non-resuscitation order is appropriate for you, and you can decline any treatment if you don't want it – but you need to make sure that the important people involved in your care know your wishes.

Looking Beyond the Now

Seeing is believing. WYSIWYG. I heard it with my own ears. I was there.

And yet, sometimes there is more to a situation than what we can see and hear before us. Sometimes our attention to the present detail prevents us from standing back to discover the pattern or meaning of what we are experiencing; sometimes our assumptions obscure other possible interpretations of the same information. The stoic philosophers asserted that it is not events themselves, but our responses to them that cause us happiness or heartache – at the prospect of the death of a beloved family member or friend, our upset may be mediated by our own sense of powerlessness or loss, or by the apparent distress of our loved one. But how clearly do we see situations in which we are deeply, emotionally immersed? What if our own assumptions and emotions impose a lens that colours our experience and understanding of what we see and hear?

The next few stories all illustrate ways in which reinterpreting the situation may give us new insights, and greater wisdom. It is not the events themselves, but the way each individual perceives them that is our best guide, and we are wise to remain aware that there can often be another way to interpret what may have seemed an essential truth.

In the Kitchen at Parties

Despite the transience of the patient-members of our hospice community, we are frequently humbled by their ability to look beyond their own needs, and to befriend and support each other. Likewise, families form fleeting support networks during the shared portions of their journey.

It was a reflection from one of these informal support groups that painted a new interpretation of our work for me.

It's a midsummer evening. The still-bright sky illuminates the hospice's Japanese garden outside the ladies' bay where four strangers are forging end-of-life friendships. Ama, a quietly dignified Japanese grandmother who married a British sailor and accompanied him to England in the 1950s; Bridget, a larger-than-life Irish matriarch who has run nursing homes in our city for many years; Patty, known as 'Nana' by her family and by all the staff, a riversider in her nineties rendered speechless by a brain tumour; and Marjorie, fondly dubbed 'the Duchess' by the staff here, who has a penchant for upmarket lingerie, fine cosmetics and expensive perfume.

Nana has been tired out by a visit from her large and enthusiastic family. She has spent the day in a wheelchair, and her adult grandchildren have wheeled her around the buildings, around the garden, around the local streets to a pizza restaurant for dinner, and then back to the hospice where, with a sigh of relief, she has been helped into bed by the nurses. Nana's right side and her speech have been affected by her brain tumour; as the swelling continues she has access to fewer words and requires more help to move, but the left half of her face remains highly expressive, usually of humour and of her fabulous sense of the absurd.

One of the things that Nana finds absurd is the amaryllis bulb that is growing opposite her, in a pot beside the Duchess's bed. This was a present from her daughter, an actress who is well known locally and is tipped for the Big Time. Presented as an Easter gift in a jaunty golden bowl, the bulb has been developing over the spring and has produced a tense, cylindrical shoot topped by a pyramidal bud, so that it now undeniably resembles an erect green penis. The Duchess either ignores or does not see this resemblance, but Nana is fascinated and endlessly amused by it, chuckling every time the Duchess asks one of the nurses to 'water my baby's flower'. As Nana's brain tumour evolves, her discretion decreases, and today she was reduced to guffaws of helpless laughter as the pot was borne aloft to the sink for watering. The nurses can barely contain their own amusement at the whole situation.

The Duchess keeps a scrapbook of newspaper cuttings charting her daughter's career, which she shows to anyone who will listen, or who cannot get away. Nana and Ama are members of that captive audience. Ama's sense of etiquette remains strongly Japanese, and she is too polite to decline invitations to look at the album. The Duchess has adopted Ama as a lady-in-waiting, and is particularly interested in her views on the art of Japanese silk painting. Her long-term lung condition now confines the Duchess to the short distance she can walk wearing her oxygen mask; the tube will not extend beyond the four-bedded bay.

Ama's bed faces across the bay to Bridget. Many years as a nurse have taught Bridget to hold her own counsel, and she recognises a quiet fellow spirit in Ama. Occasionally the pair walk together around the Japanese garden, a peaceful space that was a delightful surprise to Ama when she arrived at the hospice. Arm in arm, in silence, they point out particular points of beauty in the garden. Bridget is entertained by the gigantic golden carp in the pond; Ama is more likely to admire the juxtaposition of colours and shapes amongst the plants. Ama's Shinto spirit finds consolation in this beautiful place; Bridget's Christian soul is uplifted by being able to help her new friend.

Bridget always has a few minutes' chat with Nana's visitors, because she was once the matron of the care home where Nana lives. Bridget's breast cancer eventually forced her into retirement, but she is very touched that the family still recognise and remember her several years later. She is delighted to hear that the high standards she set in the home have been maintained by her team, and Nana hopes to be able to return there when her radiotherapy treatment is finished. To Nana, the care home is her home and the place where she wishes to live out her last days; to Bridget, it is her life's work and legacy.

Ama has been struggling with breathlessness caused by compression of her windpipe from a large oesophageal cancer. She has had radiotherapy treatment, and a special stent has been inserted into her windpipe to hold it open. She has been with us for a week, and looks very much better. Initially afraid to move away from her bed, she has been encouraged and enabled by Bridget to gather the confidence to walk outside, and next week we hope she will return home.

At our weekly team meeting yesterday we discussed each patient and, where appropriate, any of their nearest and dearest about whom we might have concerns. The relatives of the ladies in the Japanese garden bay were all up for discussion. Nana's family seem not to realise that her radiotherapy will not cure her brain tumour. Ama's husband is concerned about whether she will manage their steep stairs when she comes home. Bridget's son is worried that his mother is having a spiritual crisis: she has stopped nagging him to attend Mass. The daughter of the Duchess is starring in a West End show and cannot visit, but her comedian husband is living in the Duchess's house, visiting daily to entertain staff and patients alike, and, reports our ward sister, 'is killing us with his double entendres about that wretched plant!'

It was decided that we need to address Bridget's possible crisis of faith (chaplain to visit); Nana's son's understanding of her poor prognosis (the leader or me to have a word); Ama's domestic circumstances (occupational therapist home-assessment visit); and anyone who has not yet seen the amaryllis now wants to take a look.

This golden evening, I am on call. Although it is late, I am still here because I have agreed to meet the family of a patient who is dying, and they will arrive tonight from Australia after a twenty-six-hour journey. The chef is also working late, to make a meal for them when they arrive. He is sitting in the ward team office, where the amaryllis is under discussion.

'It's just weird and horrid!' says Amanda, one of our older nurses. 'I don't know what it's going to turn into, but today I noticed that it's starting to bend towards the light. Ugh!'

Ali, our youngest nurse, starts to giggle.

'And you' – Amanda wags her finger at Ali admonishingly – 'you shouldn't even know what we're talking about at your tender age!'

Tears are running down Ali's face. She has hiccups of laughter as she replies, 'Mandy, this is the 1980s, not the 1940s! And I *am* a nurse!'

The chef is intrigued, partly by the amaryllis and partly by the ward office banter. 'I always thought you were all so strait-laced and holy,' he murmurs, and Ali convulses into further laughter.

There is a knock at the office door, and through the glass I see the anxious face of Nana's son. The nurses snap into professional mode, and I open the door.

'Doctor, I heard you wanted to see me,' he says. 'And I need to ask you something too.'

'Yes, I'd like a chance to catch up with you,' I reply, and together we walk to the visitors' kitchen to make a cup of tea to take with us to the interview room.

In the kitchen, the comedian is holding court. Ama's husband and the husband of another patient are laughing at some comment he has just made, and then they all agree to step outside for a smoke. I make tea for Nana's son while he watches the smoker posse's retreating backs.

'Did you want to join them?' I ask. 'I'll be here for a while if you'd like a cigarette first.' He shakes his head glumly. It is as though he knows what I am about to say.

In the interview room, we sit and look at each other over the rims of our brightly coloured cups. This man, now in his seventies, is still being protected and cherished by his dying mother. He has a lifetime of coping skills to call upon, yet she has fiercely resisted letting him know how serious her illness is. Only today were we able to gain her permission to talk frankly with her family, partly to help her be less exhausted by their enthusiasm to entertain her. I wonder where to start.

'You wanted to ask something?' I say.

He puts his cup down. 'Yeah. I want to ask you if she's dying,' he says, somewhat unexpectedly. *Gosh, he must have noticed more than we thought.*

'I wonder what makes you ask that,' I begin, to feel my way into the discussion.

'Bridget did.'

'Bridget? How?'

'Mam was asleep when I arrived this evening, so I went to talk to Bridget for a while. She asked me whether I'd noticed that Mam has less energy these days, and I hadn't really. But Bridget told me that's the pattern she sees. Less energy. Then more sleepy. Then just unconscious, before people die. She's seen it so many times, and she knows Mam from before. Bridget was asking me whether the kids are ready . . .' he trails off miserably, and looks at his hands.

Wow. The network is in action. Bridget has already done my job for me.

'Well, that's what I wanted to talk to you about,' I say. 'What do you make of what Bridget said?'

'Dunno, really. Like, I've never seen anyone die. I dunno what to expect. But she definitely isn't as good as she was, is she? And her face is getting more droopy, and she can't stand up proper, and her arm's all stiff and twisted. And she can't say her words proper either. I guess it all adds up . . .' He swallows, rubs his hands together, looks up at me with pleading eyes.

I can't make this be a happy ending for him. He wants me to tell him he's wrong. But what he's noticing are the first steps on her journey.

'You're right,' I say, and he looks away, blinking. 'If you look back, how do you think she's doing now compared with a month ago?'

'Definitely worse now.'

'How about a week ago?'

He shakes his head as he says, 'Yeah, even a week ago she was better than this. I dunno why I never put it together before.'

'It's hard when it's someone you love so much. You see the person, more than what they can or can't do,' I say, and he rubs his eyes.

There is a silence while he absorbs the reality. Then he pushes his hands against his knees, straightens his back and asks, 'So, how long has she got?'

I hate this question. It's almost impossible to answer, yet people ask as though it's a calculation of change from a pound. It's not a number – it's a direction of travel, a movement over time, a tiptoe journey towards a tipping point. I give my most honest, most direct answer: I don't know exactly. But I can tell you how I estimate, and then we can guesstimate together.

I remember the leader telling Sabine about dying, and how incredulous I was as he described the process. Barely two years later, here I am using my own adapted version of those words, now with the confidence that comes from frequent practice, tempered by the caution of knowing that, for this loving son, this is a first time, and I must go gently. I must match his pace.

Together, we review the changes he has noticed: the loss of

movement, the loss of language. Then we talk about her energy levels, and how much more tired she is now than only a couple of weeks ago. Some of her tiredness may be temporary and related to her radiotherapy, but there is a clear, overarching change, and it is recognisable week by week. So we are looking at a life expectancy of weeks. Maybe enough weeks to make a month or two; not enough to reach the autumn.

He turns the teacup round and round in his hands, staring through it into a space in his mind, beginning to feel a space in his life. He is over seventy, and his mum is dying. He could be a teenager – he does not know how to bear this loss. What can I offer? I feel the inadequacy of my youth, not yet thirty and advising a man older than my father. How can I offer support? He thanks me and says he will go back to see if his mum is awake. I return to the office. The Australians have arrived. The chef has gone to make their meal. I have more bad news to break.

The smoking posse is back in the kitchen when I arrive to make a tray of beverages for the Australians. The comedian fetches a milk jug for me, while Ama's husband sympathises that I am working so late. Nana's son appears with swollen eyes and an empty cup, and the comedian pats his shoulder in solidarity. There is a sense of fellowship amongst this disparate little community of people, all assembled here by the irresistible summons at life's end. And then the comedian makes a penetrating comment.

'Last time I was in a gang like this' – he waves his hand around the room to take in his fellow visitors – 'was in the maternity hospital. A load of dads-to-be and anxious mothers, all waiting for their lasses to give birth. All comparing notes – Have her waters broken? How often are the contractions? How dilated? Is the baby's head coming down? Nipping out for a sly fag, grabbing a cuppa while the poor wife is pushing and panting . . . And all waiting for the same outcome. All watching the same process, at different stages, in different rooms. And this is the same, innit? We're all comparing progress, waiting for the same thing. And then we'll go home, and never forget you people' – he makes eye contact with me, rather than the rest of his audience, who are nodding at him – 'and you will just change the beds and get ready for the next family.'

The posse members drift out of the kitchen towards their various loved ones, and I am left alone to reflect on the comedian's fascinating declaration. I can hear him repeating it as he stumps along the corridor, paraphrasing and refining as he turns it over and polishes it into a routine he could use on stage. He has hit an essential truth. We know what the processes of both birth and death look like when they are proceeding smoothly – clear phases, predictable progression, needing companionship and encouragement but not interference: almost like watching the tide advancing up the beach. We also know when extra action is needed – when should the midwife ask the mother to push, or pant and wait? When should the process have medical interference? Likewise, our skilled and experienced nurses know when to summon a family, when to offer pain relief or treat anxiety, when simply to reassure that all is normal, that the dying is progressing as it should.

By the time I have spoken to the Australians, the sun has set and the Japanese garden is in darkness. A prowling cat on the garden wall is silhouetted against the purple sky. I walk along the corridor, now dimly lit by the nightlights, and past the ladies' bay, where a single reading lamp pierces the shadows. Bathed in the circle of light is the golden bowl and the rude amaryllis, but tonight its unseemly terminal bud has erupted into an effervescent scarlet bloom worthy of a Japanese silk painting. The flower has been born, quietly and while no one was watching, a force of nature reaching its inevitable conclusion, without help or company.

This image hovers before my eyes as I leave the building.

This 'family's eye view' of the parallel experiences at both ends of life was a great gift that has resonated with me repeatedly throughout my career, and I treasure it still. At birth and at death,

we are privileged to accompany people through moments of enormous meaning and power; moments to be remembered and retold
as family legends and, if we get the care right, to reassure and
encourage future generations as they face these great events themselves.

Please Release Me – A Side

When does a treatment that was begun to save a life become an interference that is simply prolonging death? Can a life-sustaining treatment, begun in hope, turn into a trap that binds a failing body to existence? And if so, what are the 'rules' about stopping treatment that no longer helps the person to live well?

There are so many roles in medicine that there is a home for every interest. Indeed, at medical school, which is usually a five-year university course in the UK, we play at predicting where our fellows will end up, and follow each other's professional development with interest, amusement, or even envy. My own class, which holds regular reunion weekends every five years or so, has produced a smattering of international superstars, some splendid research scientists, a galaxy of dedicated clinicians in general practice and in a variety of hospital specialties, plus several priests, a mountaineer, a philosopher and a forestry expert. We spotted the psychiatrists during our first year: eclectic or flamboyant taste in clothing, a tendency to introspection, and possessed of a vocabulary that always made conversations fizz. The surgeons were starting to declare themselves by halfway through our training: decisive and self-assured, prone to defending sometimes indefensible opinions, and often living among dismantled motor vehicles or domestic appliances that they enjoyed reassembling with variable success.

And then there are the anaesthetists. The people who can hold their nerve when the stakes are high. They often have terrifying hobbies: hang-gliding, motorbike racing, deep-sea diving. They like 'kit'. They like risk. And they often prefer their own company, in thoughtful silence or intense concentration. At work, some prefer their patients to be asleep, as in an operating theatre or an intensive care unit; some love the thrill of high-risk surgery, when an anaesthetist with a steady nerve is an essential member of the surgical team working deep inside a patient's chest, abdomen or brain; some use their intricate knowledge of nerve pathways to gravitate towards pain management; and others work in applying their knowledge of supporting patients' breathing during operations or in ICU to those people living at home whose lives can only be maintained by relying, either partly or entirely, on a ventilator to support their breathing. This is known as home ventilation.

My anaesthetist colleague from the home ventilation team asked to talk to me. This was somewhat unusual. A man of few words but enormous passion, he had not been keen to embrace the concept of palliative care, so I was intrigued about what he might want to discuss. He offered to make me coffee when I arrived at his office, so matters were clearly serious. He looked as though he would rather be a million miles away, yet he took a deep breath, and told me about his patient, Max.

The story went back ten years to when Max, then a wealthy fifty-six-year-old retired human rights lawyer, developed a swallowing problem. This very quickly turned into a life-threatening chest infection, as food was mis-swallowed into his lungs. He was admitted to hospital almost dead, and rapidly transferred to the ICU, where his breathing was supported by a ventilator while high-dose antibiotics were given to clear his chest, which they did most effectively.

But that was only the beginning of Max's problems. As the ICU staff began to wind down his ventilator to prepare him for recovery, he failed to breathe properly without it. Further tests showed that the reason for his swallowing problems was previously undiagnosed motor neurone disease, which had paralysed his throat muscles. It had also weakened his diaphragm, that mighty, dome-shaped muscle beneath our lungs that provides much of the bellows action for breathing.

Because the diagnosis of MND was only made after he was already using a ventilator, Max did not have the opportunity to discuss with his doctors whether he would choose to be ventilated – usually a decision reached after much careful consideration by each patient affected. Instead, he was in a position of having to choose whether to continue with ventilation, with a smaller machine that could be used at home and carried about with him, or to discontinue and die because his respiratory muscles would not be strong enough to support him.

One of those people who has a long MND history, I thought, thinking of Stephen Hawking. *I hope he has a supportive family . . .*

In fact, Max had been widowed in his forties and he lived alone in an elegant, isolated Georgian farmhouse. He volunteered for the Citizens Advice Bureau and his local refugee centre. His passion for justice remained undimmed, and this guided him through the crisis at diagnosis. He didn't have time to die – he had several refugee cases in mid-tribunal, and he was writing his memoirs. Instead, he accepted that he would need to live with a ventilator, and quickly decided that he could live at home, with some regular reviews by the home ventilation team, and some paid help.

Over the next ten years Max's MND had progressed very slowly, and only recently had his limb muscles become weak, rendering him bedbound and frustrated. Throughout all this time he had been fed via a PEG tube, a small plastic tube permanently inserted through his abdominal wall, down which liquid food was dripped directly into his stomach overnight using a little pump. He was well-nourished, he was awake and alert, and until a few weeks previously he was driving his car, managing his ventilator, typing his refugee asylum applications and running his own home. Now he is confined to his bed or a reclining chair, with twenty-four-hour nursing support at home.

Ah, it's a hospice referral . . . No, it's not.

My colleague explains that Max now considers that his useful life is over. He has no partner or children to live for, and he can no longer type, so he cannot work, and nor can he communicate using the 'lightwriter' machine that has served him in place of speech so well for a decade. So he wishes to discontinue using his ventilator. He perceives, with a lawyer's clarity, that he has a right to decline treatment, and so he has a right to ask for his ventilator to be discontinued. He cannot do this for himself, because his arms are too weak to manage the switches. Besides, when the machine is switched off, he will experience profound breathlessness before he loses consciousness. He has asked the home ventilation nurse for advice.

So that's why I'm here.

Almost. There's another part of this story. My colleague has looked after Max throughout those ten years, initially at clinics and later by visiting him at home. They have enjoyed each other's intellect and humour; they have discussed politics and fine wine. This is no longer simply a doctor–patient relationship – this is a friendship. And my colleague is distressed, both by the discomfort that his patient-friend may have to face, and by his own role in it.

Here is the challenge of working as a liaison specialist in hospital palliative care. Max will remain the patient of his own GP and of my colleague. I will offer advice and expertise which Max's medical team will consider. Only if I admit Max to a hospice bed will he become 'my' patient, and even then I always liaise carefully with a team that has known a patient well over many years. Despite the fact that this consultation is about Max, it is also about the home ventilation team, who are fond of him. I am being invited to advise on managing Max, but must weigh how I approach that advice with consideration of the other clinicians, those flesh-and-blood people who are so deeply involved in his care. They must have managed ventilator withdrawal many times before, so it is a mark of their personal involvement in Max's care that they are seeking external advice. This is an honour; it is also a first, and I hope it might create a precedent that will allow palliative care team involvement in the care of other patients who might benefit. So as well as an honour, it is a test.

First, the ethical considerations. Is withdrawal of treatment that results in Max's death the same as killing him? Well, if he lived at a time or in a country without access to ventilation, he would have died of his initial chest infection; we would not have said he died of 'not being ventilated'. If he had exercised his right not to be ventilated when his MND made him unable to support himself unaided, we would have said that he was dying of respiratory failure caused by MND. The fact that he has accepted ventilation for ten years does not change the fact that ventilation is an invasive treatment, and that he has a right to decline it at any time and for any reason.

However, he has recently had a dramatic escalation of the weakness in his arms and legs, that has completely changed his independence and his quality of life. This is a shocking change. Just as he initially came to terms with loss of eating, loss of speech, and the need for a ventilator (a triad that might make anyone feel despondent about their future), and has flourished despite those adversities, might he also now find that he is able to adjust to this new lifestyle? Is he depressed? Is he anxious? Does he feel that he has options? My colleague and I discuss whether Max might waive his right to stop ventilation for a few weeks, to give him a chance to discover whether living like this continues to feel as intolerable as he currently considers it. We agree that it is ethically and legally permissible to stop ventilation, but that we are also ethically obliged to ensure that Max is in the right state of mind to make such an irrevocable decision.

We also agree that, when and if Max decides to discontinue ventilation, he will need careful management of his breathlessness if he is to die comfortably. Usually, when people die of conditions where their lungs fail supply the amount of air they need, this breathing failure happens gradually. As it does so, the levels of oxygen in the blood drop, reducing the person's awareness and thinking, and the carbon dioxide levels in their blood rise, causing sleepiness. This subtle change of gas levels dissolved in the blood causes gradual loss of consciousness. It may also cause a sense of 'air hunger', or sometimes headaches, that can be managed with low doses of morphine-like drugs and sedatives, so that there is little or no breathlessness as breathing, and life, ebb away naturally.

Simply switching a ventilator from 'on' to 'off' is quite a different proposition. As soon as the ventilator ceases, an alert but paralysed patient will feel an urge to breathe and yet be unable to do so. They will have a sense of suffocating, and this will be terrifying. To prevent both breathlessness and terror, I suggest that we will need to work with Max to establish what dose of sedative allows him to sleep through a short trial of switching off his ventilator, using a painless fingertip probe that can tell us when his oxygen levels have dropped beyond the point that would normally waken someone to fight their breathlessness.

By explaining the plan to Max this week, my colleague can assure him that whilst we will not deny his request to turn off his ventilator, we will give him some time to experience living this new, more restricted life while we experiment to find the right dose of sedative. We can then be sure that, when and if the time comes to turn off the ventilator, he will remain asleep and comfortable as his breathing fails. We can plan a few overnight admissions to hospital, during which we can try a range of sedative drug doses. Once he is fully asleep, we can switch off his ventilator and test his oxygen levels, observing him closely for any signs of distress at the same time. If he wakens or becomes distressed, we will recommence the ventilator immediately, and note that the drug dose was too low. This will help us to choose a better dose next time, until we find the right dose to prevent breathlessness.

Then, if Max is still certain that he wishes to turn off his ventilator, he can choose a date to do so, and my colleague and a home ventilation team nurse will do the honours at his home, as is his wish.

Medical ethics can be an interesting challenge. We are obliged to work within the law at all times, and our patients trust us to do so. There is a clear difference between giving a drug at a dose that will suppress breathing, thus killing the patient (illegal in the UK), and giving the same drug at a dose that will suppress breathlessness, thus allowing the patient to be free from distress while their breathing fails (good clinical practice in any jurisdiction). Max is a lawyer; he will appreciate the nuance, and also the need to define the right doses of the right drugs in advance, both for his own comfort and for the legal circumspection of his medical team.

My colleague's coffee has gone cold. His shoulders, previously hunched with unhappy anticipation, are relaxed. He smiles, and says, 'Thanks.' He shifts in his chair, looking awkward, rubs his beard and continues, 'That was unexpectedly helpful. I knew the law and the ethics, but now it's a clear set of options. It was helpful to talk it through.' I assure him, with relief, that I feel honoured to have been consulted and that I'll be happy to discuss Max's care again, because it's hard when a patient becomes a friend, and we need to look after each other if we are to remain able to help our other patients.

'I don't know how you do your job,' he says as I rise to leave. 'All that dying all the time.'

I look through the office door to the ICU entrance, where lives are hanging by medically managed threads. I couldn't do his job either.

I shake my head and smile. We shake hands. We will go on to work together in the future, supporting each other in situations too challenging to imagine today. But today we don't know that, we only know that we have found common ground and a safe place to talk about one of the toughest parts of our job: making friends with patients who are making friends with death.

Please Release Me – B Side

Many people fear the possibility of unbearable suffering as a consequence of illness or accident. Some states around the world have legalised the practice of euthanasia or of assisted suicide, in the hope that this will both reduce fear of an intolerable future for the many and provide an early death as an alternative to suffering for the few. This is based on humanitarian principles and utilitarian ethics.

And yet, even the most carefully-thought-through changes can have perverse and unintended consequences.

'They didn't mean to frighten me. I think they thought it was a comfort. But it was every day, every ward round, they told me that if I want to, I can choose to die . . .' Ujjal is explaining why he recently ran away from a hospital in his adopted home town in the Netherlands and returned to live with his mother in England, bringing his toddler and his Dutch wife with him.

Having studied languages at university, Ujjal found work with an oil company based in Rotterdam. As a rising star in the company's management training programme he had a department of many people to manage by the age of thirty, and when he married a fellow employee there was a wonderful Sikh wedding in the British town where he grew up, at which the newlyweds introduced their Dutch and British families to each other amidst the shared national enthusiasms of good food, good music and an excellent party.

Their daughter, Tabitha, was born eighteen months later. As a grandchild of two nations she was intended to grow up bilingual, so Ujjal spoke to her always in English, whilst her mama always spoke Dutch. When Tabitha was a year old, Ujjal developed abdominal swelling and a change in bowel habit. He booked an appointment with his GP. This was the point at which his nightmare began.

The GP found a large tumour in Ujjal's rectum, and referred him for treatment. Ujjal's company medical insurance ensured that he saw the best doctors in the Netherlands. They diagnosed a sarcoma of the rectum, a very rare cancer that can be cured by complete surgical removal, provided it has not already spread. Ujjal's rectum, lower bowel and bladder were removed. A false bladder was made using a portion of his intestines. He had a bag on his belly to collect his urine and another to collect his faeces. He felt lucky to be alive.

But not for long. The wound in his lower abdomen never fully recovered after his surgery. He developed an oozing sore at one end of it that wept smelly pus. Antibiotics seemed to make no difference. Then he noticed that the same smelly ooze was staining his underwear; somehow, the pus was leaking through a minute crack in the skin behind his scrotum. Further scans, more surgery. A wine-cork-sized tumour in his pelvis was removed, and radiotherapy followed to kill any unseen cells that were left behind. The ooze continued.

Then one day, the smell of the skin ooze changed. There were faeces in the discharge. More scans, more surgery. The lower part of Ujjal's bowel had shrivelled up in reaction to the radiotherapy, and burst. His pelvis was filled with excrement, germs swarmed into his bloodstream, he had unbearable abdominal pain. He passed out on the ward and woke up in the intensive care unit after further surgery, now with a third bag on his belly to collect discharge from the damaged bowels. But still the ooze continued.

A week after the latest surgery, the softly spoken and very kind professor of surgery came to sit beside Ujjal's ICU bed. He asked Ujjal how he was feeling, and offered to speak English if Ujjal preferred. They continued in Dutch, although the professor explained medical expressions in English for him. He told Ujjal that although the surgery had cleaned his pelvis and removed the damaged bowel to stop the leak of faeces and germs, he still had some tumour in his pelvis, and that this would continue to grow. At the moment the cancer was hollow, like a tennis ball, and germs were growing inside, making a filling of pus. Every now and then the pressure built up and the pus leaked out, either through his abdominal wound or down through his skin under his bottom. This was very unfortunate, but there was no further surgery that would help. Did he understand?

Ujjal understood. He had cancer, and it could not be cured. But he was alive, and he had a daughter who needed her daddy and a wife who needed her husband. And he needed to go home to spend whatever time he could with them.

The professor nodded. 'The difficult thing is,' he said, 'that the cancer will keep on growing. It will make more pressure, and this will make more pain and more leakage of pus. It will become more smelly, and the skin will become very sore. The wounds will eventually become damaged, and begin to break down. Do you understand?'

Ujjal understood. He was going to become more sore and more smelly. It could start any time. So the sooner he got home, the better.

The professor looked sad, as though it was he himself who had the pain. He said, very carefully, 'Many people would not wish to live in that state.'

Ujjal agreed that he did not wish to live in that state: this was not his choice. But if the only way to live was in that state, he wanted to do so at home.

The professor paused before saying, 'Of course, you do have a choice.'

In what way, Ujjal wondered, could he have any choice.

'Here in the Netherlands, there is an extra choice for you. If you would not like to live like that, then we have the euthanasia. Do you understand?'

Ujjal did. He understood that he could choose to die now or die later.

The professor nodded. 'Any time it is too much to bear, you have that choice. Would you like to think about that, and then one of my colleagues can come and talk to you to see what you have decided.'

'No,' Ujjal had replied. 'I don't need to think about it. I want to go home.'

'Of course, the nursing care you will need is very intensive, for the wounds and the hygiene,' said the professor. 'I am not at all sure that this kind of care can be given at home. I will leave you now to think over our discussion.' He rose from his chair, beamed his kind smile at Ujjal, and left the ICU.

Ujjal reflected. He thought the professor had managed that difficult topic very well. In his professional role Ujjal trained people to broach difficult topics of conversation, and he gave the prof full marks. He knew now that he could choose to die if living got too tough. He understood how that thought might be a comfort to someone else. But he also knew that his heart lay at home, and that even if he needed to bring his mum from England to help with Tabitha, home was where he wanted to be. Tomorrow he would begin planning his discharge from hospital.

The next day, the nurses came to change the dressings over the scar from the emergency surgery Ujjal could not remember, and to examine the new, pouting lip-like rings of flesh where his damaged bowel now joined the skin on his belly, emptying foul bowel products into plastic bags. The nurses brought a young doctor, a member of the surgery team, who wanted to check how the wounds were healing. She seemed pleased by the pink and fleshy lips of the stomata, and the line of stitches down the wound that stretched from Ujjal's pubis to the top of his abdomen.

The nurses completed their task and withdrew; the surgeon sat down beside Ujjal. 'It was a big operation, you know,' she said, 'because we needed to clean all the mess inside. I'm sorry you needed another bag, but there was a section of intestine that seemed very damaged, and we didn't dare join the ends together in case it leaked and made you so sick again.'

Ujjal was tired. He wasn't sure he wanted to talk about his insides today. But the young surgeon continued, in a voice that was kind and concerned. 'It will become difficult for you in the future if the leakage continues. We will try to manage any pain you may have. But if you prefer not to endure the progress of the illness, we have colleagues who will help you with euthanasia. You will qualify because of the extent of the disease you have. We will be able to sign the forms to give permission. You only have to ask . . .'

Ujjal rested his head in the pillow and closed his eyes. He wanted to talk about going home. He would ask the nurses later.

By the end of the next week, Ujjal's IV drips were down, he was eating small meals, and his wounds were healing. His bags were functioning, and he was moved from ICU to a surgery ward to continue to recuperate.

Now, each day followed the same pattern: early breakfast, then managing his stoma bags himself, as a matter of principle, despite offers of help from the nurses; a shower – oh, the joy of a shower after so many days of bed baths – and changing his sweaty pyjamas; a nap; lunch; a visit from a friend, or possibly from Tabitha with Mama; another nap; and at the end of the afternoon the surgeons' ward round to inspect wounds, palpate abdomens, plan further treatment or give permission to go home. Every day he heard the doctors discuss progress with his neighbours: one who may need physiotherapy, another who needed an X-ray, someone who was ready to walk on stairs, the person who was well enough to go home. At Ujjal's bed, the doctors were always so kind. They asked about Tabitha, they asked about his pain, they asked about the ooze. They asked whether he had any worries. And they reminded him that if it got too hard to bear, he could talk to them about euthanasia. Then they moved on.

Ujjal began to dread the ward rounds, to fear the relentless cheer of benevolent voices that offered antibiotics to some, physiotherapy to others, and death to him, like items on a treatment menu. He began to realise that the kind doctors were fearful for him. They could envisage further deterioration in his condition, a deterioration that they considered hopeless, undignified, horrifying; a deterioration that would be worse than being dead. Ujjal began to perceive the sunny, six-bed bay as a prison from which death was the only escape. He knew he had to leave.

The professor was brought to reason with him; Ujjal's wife was sent for too. The prof explained to them both that Ujjal had very delicate wounds; some infection that could not be eradicated because the bowel was still leaking internally; tumour still growing, outstripping its own blood supply, dying in the centre and turning to mushy ooze that leaked from Ujjal's broken wounds. This is not because you are not a clean person, he reassured him with great warmth and empathy, it is the way the tumour behaves. It makes the smell and the oozing discharge no matter how many times you bathe. Many people would prefer not to live in this condition . . .

Ujjal demanded his bag and his belongings. He insisted on being driven home by his wife, and then he telephoned his mother in England and asked to borrow the money for the boat trip to return to her house. Within a week he was resident in his mother's spare bedroom, while Tabitha and her mama slept in the room next door in old bunk beds used by Ujjal and his sister as children. This is where his mother's GP came to visit him, and where he was referred to our hospice.

Our hospice outreach nurse visited Ujjal at home, and came back to discuss how we might be able to help. She described his needs under our usual 'Physical', 'Emotional', 'Social' and 'Spiritual' headings. Physically, Ujjal was thin and pale, dehydrated but too nauseated to drink much. He had intermittent abdominal pain, and the skin of his scrotum was becoming sore because of his frequent washing of the smelly ooze. Emotionally, he was relieved to be out of the reach of further offers of help to die, however kindly intended, but he was anxious about what might happen to make his life the 'worse than death' scenario clearly anticipated by the Dutch doctors. Socially, the house was too small for Ujjal, his wife, their active toddler, his mother and the many friends who came to visit daily. Tabitha was confused by the regional English accent, clinging to her mama and speaking only in Dutch. The position of Ujjal's bed made nursing care difficult. Spiritually, he swung between two extremes. Sometimes he was buoyed by his hope to remain alive long enough to see Tabitha start school; bargaining with a God he was not sure he believed in caused him to play down his pain in an effort to 'win points'. At other times he wondered whether he had been a coward to run away; whether, in failing to embrace euthanasia while his quality of life was still tolerable, he had brought sadness and an inescapable burden on the people he loved.

Ujjal was admitted to a single room at the hospice the next day. A day-bed in the room was made up for his wife, and we borrowed a travel cot for Tabitha. In effect, they took up residence while we considered how best to support Ujjal's decision to live with his most beloved women for the rest of his foreshortened life. Gradually we acquired more background information, and the Dutch doctors were wonderfully helpful in sending English summaries of their records, scans and surgery notes.

Ujjal was enthusiastic to try any experiment that might improve his wellbeing. Thus, we devised ways to use tampons to collect the pus from the wound in his bottom; we used drugs to alter the consistency of his faeces to reduce leakage; we used special wound dressings to contain and reduce the smelly ooze. Although the cancer mass in his pelvis was growing, we used a spinal line to numb the pain – the usual intolerable side-effect of loss of bowel and bladder control was already solved by the system of collection bags since his surgery. Ujjal adapted to wheelchair mobility, taking Tabitha for rides around the hospice and grounds. They both took a mid-afternoon snooze, for which we were all grateful – Tabitha was a delightful bundle of noisy energy, and the respite was vital for everyone.

Today Ujjal is explaining to Emma, one of our trainee doctors, about the Dutch healthcare system. He knows that he was expertly managed throughout his illness, by knowledgeable, competent, kind practitioners in the Netherlands. He appreciates the expertise of the surgery and ICU teams who, despite the challenges, have certainly extended his life. His only criticism is that there was a subtle, entirely unintended nuance in every consultation once his cancer began to spread. In the end, this nuance was too frightening to tolerate.

The possibility of allowing euthanasia, without prosecuting doctors who follow a strict set of rules, is permitted in the Netherlands to provide a legal escape route from unbearable suffering towards the end of life, and Ujjal had admired the Dutch pragmatism that enabled this practice. Yet once the possibility of euthanasia was raised for him, he found that he was afraid to admit to new symptoms, in case euthanasia rather than symptom management was recommended. His conversations with his doctors developed a new tone: their sense of helplessness in the face of his symptoms, and hopelessness at his prognosis, communicated itself to him. He perceived a preference to control the uncertainty of his disease progression by accelerating his death. Ujjal ran away from that certain, controlled dying to live with the hope of uncertainty. It was a compromise that might break his body, yet save his sanity. He had experienced an unintended and chilling consequence of an entirely humanitarian change in legislation.

Ujjal lived with us for two months. Tabitha developed a local English accent and demonstrated enormous promise as a future gymnast over that period: all the furniture in the room required repair or replacement after her departure.

Ujjal's cancer eventually obstructed his kidneys, and he became comatose over a few days before dying very quietly while Tabitha was running and laughing in the garden outside his room.

She and her mother returned to the Netherlands.

We don't know whether Tabitha is still bilingual.

This possibility of unintended pressure is a dilemma currently confronting healthcare systems across the world. Once the euthanasia genie is out of the bottle, you must be careful what you wish for.

Travel Plans

It seems that the sense of approaching departure is apparent to many people as their illness progresses. Sometimes the metaphor of leave-taking is the only way the approach of death can be discussed. Over the years I have met people who perplexedly search for their passports, ask their baffled loved ones to check their tickets, put random items into bags for the journey. I have learned not to confront the 'confusion', but to join in the conversation where the patient is, and through it to reach, discuss and comfort their sense of imminent departure.

Sanjeev and Arya have been married for 'sixty-odd' years, he announces, adding, 'I'd better get that number right when she's here!' Sanjeev has heart failure. After a healthy old age, he had a heart attack last year at the age of eighty-eight, and his weakened heart cannot now support any vigorous activity, for example talking at the same time as walking. He has been admitted to hospital from the cardiology clinic, because his blood tests show that his kidneys are starting to fail. Bed rest and adjustment of his medications are required.

Arya brings food from home. The delicious smell wafts along the ward, and the other patients in Sanjeev's bay ask if they can give her an order. Arya smiles and tells them she will bring them all a snack tomorrow.

After dark, it's a busy night in that small bay. One of the men has a cardiac arrest. His heart monitor sounds an alarm and the ward team, along with a doctor from the CCU (coronary care unit), spring into action. There is commotion, clipped medical phrases, running feet, the 'Thud!' of a defibrillator. The heart restarts; the patient is wheeled off to CCU on his bed, leaving a space in the six-bedded bay. The other patients are wide awake, shaken.

'Like telly,' observes one of them.

'I'm glad I'm going home tomorrow,' says another.

'Indeed,' agrees Sanjeev. 'I also will be going home tomorrow.' The other men are surprised; they were anticipating several days of tasty snacks from Arya while Sanjeev was on bed rest.

'Where's home for you then, mate?' asks a stocky, tattooed man who is having his high blood pressure treated.

Sanjeev considers this question. 'It's near Delhi,' he says, naming a small town in which he spent his childhood before coming to Britain for his education. 'Perhaps you know it?' The tattooed man says he's never been to India. Sanjeev looks perplexed. 'It's only round the corner. Are you silly?'

A nurse brings in a tray of milky drinks and says, 'OK, chaps, your pal is doing fine. Sorry we woke you with all the clamour. Who'd like a warm drink?' Three of the men ask for malted milk, one for tea, and Sanjeev for chai. He is put out when the nurse says there is no chai.

'No chai!' he grumbles. 'What kind of hotel is this?' He hauls his swollen legs over the edge of his bed and stands up. He asks the nurse, 'Madam, if you would kindly reach my suitcase for me,' and begins to retrieve his clothes from his bedside locker. Then he sits down and begins to search through his wallet; dissatisfied, he rummages in the locker drawer, then in his toilet bag, then back to his wallet.

'Sanjeev, are you looking for something?' asks the nurse.

Sanjeev looks at her anxiously. 'I seem to have mislaid my tickets, madam, although I can assure you that they are all in order. Do you need to see them now, or might I show them later?'

The nurse asks him to get back into bed, and he asks her what time the train will arrive in Delhi. And suddenly she understands.

'We won't arrive until morning, sir,' she says, realising that she has somehow become transformed into a railway official in his mind. 'We're asking all passengers to make themselves comfortable, and I will call you in plenty of time. Now, can I assist you back to bed?'

Sanjeev agrees politely, and she helps him to climb back onto his bed ('High bunks in here!' he grumbles) and settles him down. She asks if anyone will be meeting him off the train.

'My parents,' Sanjeev smiles. 'It's been so long since I saw them.'

The nurse is an experienced night-shift worker. She leaves a dim light on by Sanjeev's bed, and draws his curtain slightly to screen it from the other 'passengers', because she knows that darkness compounds disorientation, and that being able to see familiar objects is calming. Then she returns to the nurses' station and calls the doctor. She reports that her patient is delirious and disorientated in time and place, and believes he is in India, travelling to meet his parents. She asks whether she should call Sanjeev's wife.

The doctor is very young. To have a job in this institution, she must be academically very bright. She is in the CCU, where she has just finished stabilising Sanjeev's erstwhile room-mate.

'Why would we disturb his wife?' she asks. 'We need to find out why he's delirious, and treat him. I'll come and listen to his chest and take some blood for tests. Please will you repeat his observations while I'm on my way?'

The nurse goes back to Sanjeev, who is once again fumbling in his wallet for tickets. 'Please don't worry about your tickets, sir, I have them safely in my office,' she says.

Sanjeev submits to having his temperature, pulse and blood pressure measured, seeming to think this is an extended service on the railway, and then says, 'Thank you, Mummy.'

The nurse sits down on the bedside chair, and asks, 'Do you wish your mummy was here?' He looks puzzled, so she shows him her uniform, the clip-watch hanging from her dress, the pocket of pens, to help him recognise that she is a nurse. 'What would you say to your mummy if she was here?' she asks him gently, and Sanjeev tells her, 'I have missed you, Mummy. I am so glad to be coming home.'

The nurse squeezes his hand. 'And she must miss you, Sanjeev. She will be so glad to see you.'

Sanjeev closes his eyes and dozes off. The nurse returns to her station and phones Arya, asking her to come to the hospital as soon as she can.

The young doctor arrives, looking flustered from her busy shift. The nurse produces Sanjeev's case notes, summarises his day from admission to becoming disoriented, and reports that his temperature, pulse and blood pressure are all normal. The doctor goes to examine Sanjeev, and the nurse advises, 'If he believes you're railway staff, just tell him you're the railway doctor and that it's all part of a new service.' The doctor stares at her blankly, and the nurse goes on, 'If you challenge his perception of reality he'll simply become upset and anxious. Let's keep him calm. When his wife arrives, we can try to reorientate him.'

'But why have you called his wife?' asks the doctor.

'Because he thinks he's on his way home to his mother,' says the nurse's Voice of Wisdom, 'and in my clinical experience, that's a sign that he may be dying. I'd rather call his wife for a false alarm than not heed his message.'

The doctor goes off to assess Sanjeev while the nurse goes back to her rounds of observations, answering patient buzzers and giving out medications. They meet back at the nurses' station, where the doctor is labelling the vials of blood she has just taken from Sanjeev and calling the labs to ask for urgent tests. 'His chest is clear,' she says, 'but he has an odd tremor and his ECG changes make me wonder whether his kidneys are deteriorating. What's his resuscitation status?'

The nurse reports that Sanjeev and his wife are both aware that Sanjeev's heart is damaged beyond repair, and that if it should fail, or stop beating, resuscitation would not succeed. 'The consultant has discussed it, and they agree with him. There's a Do Not Attempt Cardio-Pulmonary Resuscitation order in his notes,' the nurse reports. The case notes record the important conversation between the consultant and the couple, when he explained to them that CPR could not succeed and that a DNACPR order would protect Sanjeev from 'unhelpful interference' if his heart became too weak to support him. The conversation took place about six months ago, and is recorded in the consultant's bold, pointy handwriting. He has helpfully included the exact words he used to explain the situation, and the couple's response: '*Patient and wife understand. They would not wish CPR to be his terminal event. They are keen to avoid "medical interference". DNACPR form completed. GP notified.*'

The ward doorbell sounds, and Arya arrives. The nurse greets her and explains that Sanjeev is muddled and thinks he is on a train to Delhi. She hopes that seeing Arya will help him to feel calm and safe. 'He thinks he's going to meet his parents,' she says, 'and he mistook me for his mother. Would you like to come and see him? The doctor has examined him and is sending off some blood tests, and she'll let you know as soon as we get some results.'

Arya follows the nurse into the dimly lit bay, and approaches her husband.

'Arya!' He recognises her immediately. 'What are you doing here? Who is looking after our babies?'

Arya is taken aback, but the nurse is ready. 'The babies are with an expert nanny, Sanjeev, and Arya has explained exactly how they must be cared for. Now, can I get you both a cup of tea? I must apologise that there is no chai.'

By now, dawn is breaking. Sanjeev points to the window and says, 'We are nearly there, Arya. Hurry, we must dress the babies and get ready to show them to Mummy.' He starts to climb out of his bed. The doctor appears at this moment, to tell Sanjeev and Arya that she has the lab results and wishes to discuss them. She tries to persuade Sanjeev to get back into bed, but he is adamant that he must wash, dress and prepare his paperwork for arrival in Delhi. The doctor returns to the nurses' station for back-up.

Backup, it transpires, is available in the form of the new shift of nurses, just getting their handover from the night staff. I am there too, having come in early to review a patient's pain before I go to a meeting. The night nurse briefly summarises Sanjeev's confusion journey: triggered by the sudden awakening during the cardiac arrest event, via briefly thinking that the ward was a hotel, to his fixed belief that he is on the train home to his parents in Delhi, parents who have been dead for forty years. The doctor adds that Sanjeev's blood tests show that his kidneys have failed completely, so he has rising potassium levels in his blood that put him at risk of abnormal heart rhythms, even cardiac arrest. She suggests that he should have treatment to lower the potassium, and that he may need kidney dialysis. His delirium is related to the speed at which his kidneys have failed.

I ask whether Sanjeev would want dialysis. The young doctor looks perplexed. 'He *needs* dialysis,' she says.

I agree that if Sanjeev is to survive long-term, he probably needs dialysis. 'But is that what he wants?' I ask. 'He has already told his consultant that he doesn't want to be messed around, that he understands that he will eventually die from his heart failure. Perhaps this is the way his dying will happen – from kidney failure.' The young doctor blinks tiredly back at me, and I say, 'You need a coffee; Sanjeev needs a decision. Shall we have a cuppa with Sanjeev and his wife, and see what's the best thing to do?'

The weary doctor has another hour before her shift will end, and the nurses can see that she is near the end of her tether. This is a big decision, a medical decision, in which the patient's views must be considered. But can Sanjeev really express a considered opinion while he believes he is on a train in another continent? I have participated in many, many of these conversations, and I explain that we must explore the patient's views as far as we can, then we will call Sanjeev's consultant to make the medical decision.

The doctor and I take our cups of coffee to Sanjeev's bedside. The young doctor is concerned that this will look unprofessional, and I reassure her that, on the contrary, it gives the message that we are prepared to sit and spend time with the couple, and in his confusion Sanjeev needs such 'body language' signals to feel secure. I introduce myself, and then ask Sanjeev how things are going.

'I need to get ready. We are nearly there,' he says. I reply that I understand that all his paperwork is in order, and that I can help Arya to pack his bag if there is any need to hurry. I ask him to tell me about his heart condition. 'Oh, my old ticker. It gives me no trouble.' Arya looks startled, but he continues, 'It's getting old, like me. I can't hurry and my legs swell up, but it gives me no pain. Just tiredness. I am getting so tired . . .' It is the young doctor's turn to look surprised; despite being on an Indian train, Sanjeev is able to discuss his heart condition.

'What will happen to your heart in the future?' I ask him.

Sanjeev looks at Arya, and says, 'Well, it will be the death of me, certainly. We both know this. We both know that the re-suscitation team cannot save me. This I must tell my parents. I am taking Arya to tell them.'

'If there were treatments that might help you to live longer, Sanjeev, would you want to do that?' I ask.

Sanjeev considers. He looks at Arya again. He says, 'I have had a very long life. I have done very many things. I have been most fortunate. I have had a very happy marriage and two sons.' He smiles at Arya. 'But life is not everything if weakness overtakes you. I am overtaken by weakness; I will never be strong again. What use is it to prolong living in a useless way? Is there a treat-ment to make me strong? No. Is there a treatment to make me young? No. Can you make me fit and strong? No, you cannot, and this we must accept. So living longer is not a good thing if I live like an invalid.'

The young doctor sips her coffee, pensive and pale. When Sanjeev takes a sip of his tea, the doctor looks concerned and whispers, 'Fluid balance.' Nodding to her, to show that I have heard her, I ask Arya, 'Is this something you've discussed before? Do you talk about these things together?'

'We talked a lot after the heart consultant, Dr Abel, told us about the resuscitation problem,' Arya replies, keeping her gaze on Sanjeev as she speaks, 'and we both agree this. Being alive but not living well, that is not good. We were very grateful that Dr Abel was so honest with us. Sanjeev explained it to our sons, and we have arranged everything. When Sanjeev dies . . .' she swallows, and continues. 'When that happens, I will go to live with our younger son. He is near. I will feel near Sanjeev until it is my turn.'

There is a pause. Drinks are sipped. There is a sense of togetherness around the bed. Sounds of morning activity begin in the bay: footsteps, medicines trolley, names checked and drugs administered, the hum of the blood pressure monitor.

'Sanjeev, Arya, the problem we have today is this –' I begin.

'Have we missed the station?!' asks Sanjeev, sharply. 'Where are my tickets?'

'No, there's still quite a journey,' I say. 'It's a medical problem, not a travel problem. Can I ask you about this medical problem?'

'Indeed,' says Sanjeev.

'Well,' I say, 'it seems that your heart condition has now caused your kidneys to stop working properly. That might be quite serious.' I pause. Arya nods.

Sanjeev asks, 'How serious?'

'Serious enough to shorten your life,' I say, deliberately calmly and clearly.

'How short?' he asks. 'Where are my tickets?'

'Perhaps as short as days with no treatment,' I say.

He looks at me, looks at Arya, and then back at me. 'Well, then,' he announces, 'we must get home from India as soon as possible.'

'Do you mean go home for treatment?' I ask.

He raises his hand, shakes his head, and says, 'No, no, no, no. Arya and I have discussed this many times. I wish to die in our own home. No more hospital carry-on. No machines. No "beep-beep" nonsense. At home. With my parents. As we planned.'

'Parents?' I say, and he considers before saying, 'Are you trying to catch me out? I am in my eighties. My parents were cremated in India many years ago. I am going to pay my respects.'

'I'm sorry, Sanjeev. Perhaps I misheard you. I thought you said you wanted to be with your parents when you die.'

'Silly-silly,' he pats my hand. 'I am always with my parents, I carry them in my heart. I want to be at home with my family. Look at my lovely wife, doctor. She knows how to care for me. Send me home to her.'

I tell him that I will do my best, then the young doctor and I withdraw to call Sanjeev's consultant. He knows the couple well, and asks me whether I think Sanjeev has the capacity to make a decision about whether or not to have further treatment. I tell him that, despite his muddle about place and time, he is able to express very clearly his views about avoiding a 'medically compli-cated' death, views that are aligned with all the conversations his consultant has previously had with him.

Dr Abel says that haemodialysis (the filtering and purification of the blood by a machine) is an invasive procedure, and that Sanjeev may no longer be fit enough to survive it. We discuss the best way to ensure that he will not be troubled by symptoms like nausea and hiccups caused by his kidney failure; I assure Dr Abel that I can arrange for the community palliative care team to visit Sanjeev at home later today if we can arrange his discharge from hospital this morning. It is agreed. Sanjeev's son is called to provide transport; the weary junior doctor is sent home to sleep.

Sanjeev supervises his packing, and Arya collects his medicines from the hospital pharmacy. Dr Abel comes to the ward and asks him how he is. Sanjeev begins to look for his tickets once more, and the consultant says that tickets are not required, he is an honoured guest. Sanjeev beams at the nurses as a porter wheels him along the ward on his way to the car park.

The community palliative care team calls me the following morning. Sanjeev continued to look for his tickets at home before agreeing to get into bed. His sons and Arya around him, he settled to sleep, with a weary Arya cuddled up beside him. And when she woke up, Sanjeev was no longer breathing.

'He has arrived at his destination,' Arya told their sons. 'He will wait for us there.'

The writing of a non-resuscitation order is an important interaction between patient, clinician and family. It is vital that the family is aware of the order, and of its reasons, so that dispute and distress are avoided should the patient collapse. Knowing that there are plans for appropriate treatment, and also plans to avoid inappropriate or unwanted escalation, is a central part of planning end-of-life care.

With Love from Me to You

Anticipating death can enable a dying person to consider their options, and to make clear plans for what care they would like as death approaches. For some people this might mean 'Try as hard as possible to keep me alive,' but for most (and especially for any who have seen a peaceful death) it will mean 'Focus on my peace and comfort, not the length of survival.' People can discuss where they would like to be cared for at the end of life: this may be at home, or at the home of a dear one. Some may require the additional resources of a care home or hospice setting. Most people would prefer not to die in hospital, yet without a plan for 'what to do in an emergency', many find themselves bounced into hospital against their preference.

People who are found to be dying despite the best efforts of a hospital admission can only express a choice if the hospital team is clear about their outlook. Making plans ahead of time requires the sick person, their dear ones, and their medical advisers to have the courage (and the skill, for professionals) to have honest, clear conversations about what it is, and what it is not, possible to offer. Only then can a dying person and their dear ones make a well-informed choice.

It's late morning when a GP calls me from a patient's house. She has been there for an hour, and over that time the elderly patient has looked progressively less well. He has a long-standing liver condition, is known to be approaching the end of his life, and he has an Emergency Health Care Plan that makes it clear that his priority is comfort, not heroic efforts to save his life. Today he has overwhelming nausea that prevents him lying down. Can I make any suggestions for his nausea? We discuss some medical details, I offer some advice, and tell the GP that I can get there in twenty minutes.

I struggle to park at the patient's house: it is in a quiet suburb built without driveways or garages, and parked cars are crowded along the roadside. It is summer, and children are playing in the narrow, quiet street – skipping, cycling, and a game that involves chalked patterns on the road and a lot of laughter. The porch door is open, and inside, the front door is ajar. I knock and call, 'Hello! Dr Mannix here. Please may I come in?'

A tear-stained woman in incongruously cartoonish pyjamas pulls the door wide. 'Thanks for coming so quickly,' she says. 'Sorry about the PJs . . .'

Along the short hallway I can see into the kitchen, where Deidre, a local district nursing sister beloved by the palliative care team for her kind, no-nonsense approach, spots me and shouts, 'Good! Come here!' I obey. Everyone always does.

Deidre summarises in a low voice what has been happening to the patient, Walter, who is well known to her team of nurses. She tells me he is on his bed in the living room, where I will also find his two daughters (she rolls her eyes in a silent gesture of 'Expect emotion') and his lady-friend, Molly. The GP gave Walter an injection for his nausea after our phone call, and has gone off to see other patients. Walter is now feeling less nauseated, and has been able to lie down. Deidre takes me through to the living room.

The room runs the depth of the house. Silver fabric blinds on the large front windows filter bright daylight into a white glow, illuminating an elderly woman in a dressing gown and hairnet sitting in an armchair beside the window. This is Molly. Her gaze is fixed on the single bed at the back end of the room in which a pale, thin man with yellow-tinged skin and wispy white hair is lying quietly. He is propped up on a pile of pillows and is panting, eyes closed and lips pursed. He looks far older than his sixty-odd years. The young woman in pyjamas sobs on a dining chair beside the bed, and another young woman in a smart suit (which looks odd amongst the pyjama-clad family) is standing beside her, stroking her arm. Deidre introduces me, then retires to the kitchen to continue writing her notes of the morning's proceedings.

After greeting the women, I walk to the bedside and kneel down. The daughters protest that I should take the chair, but I am content here, close to the patient and also, I now realise, close to a large black-and-white collie that is lying quietly beneath Walter's bed. It's always wise to make friends with the house dog. He sniffs my hand, then eyes me with a baleful stare and shifts posture so my knees have room. This, I am told, is Sweep, Walter's companion for ten years, who is not usually allowed inside the house apart from the kitchen. He has been crying this morning, and so has been granted admittance. He took up this station close to Walter, and has not moved since.

'Hello, Walter,' I greet the weary patient. 'I'm Dr Kathryn, from the palliative care team, and I'm here to see whether we can sort out this sick feeling you've got. Do you think you can manage to talk a little bit?'

Walter opens his eyes, and I am struck by the deep, buttercup yellow of the whites, and the pale blue irises in stark contrast. He sighs and clears his throat. 'I'll try . . .'

'I can see you're very tired, Walter, so I can start by talking to your family, and you just correct us if we go wrong anywhere. OK?' I suggest, and Walter agrees.

Molly interrupts to say, 'I'm not really family,' and the daughter in the suit responds gently, 'Molly, Dad loves you, and so do we. You are a really important member of our family –' before filling up with tears. Her sister nods, too emotional to speak.

Molly blinks back her own tears, and says, 'This is why your dad loves you both so much. For your kind hearts.' *I am watching a family discovering itself.*

Over the last few months, Walter has had less energy. As his liver tests showed a continuous slow deterioration, his horizons began shrinking. He used to enjoy walking Sweep to the local park, but over the last few weeks a neighbour has been calling to exercise the dog. Getting up the stairs was becoming a struggle. The daughters suggested bringing his bed downstairs, but Walter's bathroom is upstairs, and he was unwilling to consider using urine bottles or a commode.

For the past two days, Walter has been confined to his chair in the living room, too nauseated to move. He had lost his appetite in the past couple of weeks, feeling full all the time. Yesterday he was surprised by feeling suddenly sick, and then needing to vomit. He had been astonished at how big the vomit had been – 'Caught it in the washing-up bowl, luckily,' he reported. An ever-practical man, he rinsed out the bowl, found a clean bucket and retired to his armchair, where Molly found him stranded by nausea when she arrived to make their lunch.

In response to Molly's SOS, one daughter drove across the country straight away (bearing her own daughter's pyjamas), while the other booked a next-day flight. PJ daughter and Molly persuaded Walter that he would sleep better in his bed, and the neighbours helped them move it downstairs. Walter was embarrassed to find himself 'as weak as a kitten' and in need of help to get ready for bed. Molly sat up in the armchair until he was asleep, then went home for her essentials and returned to stay the night.

The household was startled awake by Walter loudly retching and moaning at around 5 a.m. They sat with him, mopping his face with cool wet cloths and rinsing the bucket as he tried, but failed, to bring up any vomit. They rang for a doctor at 8 a.m., suit daughter arrived from the airport around nine, and the doctor came at ten, along with the district nurse. This is why Molly and one daughter are still in their nightwear. They have not left Walter's side since early morning. I guess that nobody has eaten either.

'Have you been having hiccups, Walter?' I ask him.

'Stupendous hiccups!' he replies, looking curious.

Ah, it's starting to make sense . . . This constellation of symptoms – fullness after eating very little, hiccups, sudden nausea relieved by large-volume vomits – all adds up to a problem with the stomach emptying effectively. The human stomach can hold a surprising volume (just think about what we might ask it to hold at Christmas or other festive occasions), and if it doesn't empty properly, initially it just stretches, tickling the local nerves and causing hiccups. Finally, when it is just too full to take any more, there is a sudden feeling of 'I'm going to be sick!' and then a spectacularly large vomit, which empties the stomach, relieves all the symptoms, and lets the cycle start again.

Now that his nausea has been relieved by the drug given by his GP, an exhausted Walter is falling asleep. I suggest to Molly and PJ daughter that they might take the opportunity to get dressed while I examine Walter, and they gratefully head upstairs. Suit daughter looks restless and anxious. She has been awake for hours, has flown the length of the country, and has had no break-fast. She takes the chance to escape to the kitchen for tea and toast while Deidre and I take a closer look at Walter. Deidre comments that she doesn't take sugar, and suit daughter smiles and takes everyone's order for a cuppa.

Walter's skin glows an almost luminous yellow in the filtered daylight. He is wasted, with protruding cheekbones and teeth that look too big for his mouth. His skin is waxy and moist; his muscles hang loose from his bones. His ribs protrude and his tummy is swollen. Beneath the blanket, his legs are also swollen, their skin stretched shiny and tight. This is advanced liver failure.

Deidre inspects Walter's buttocks and heels, areas where skin damage is common in bedbound patients. Walter, of course, was still up and about yesterday, and his skin is fine. Deidre's team will keep it that way. She goes out to her car to collect some items that will help to protect Walter's skin. Children's laughter fills the air momentarily as the door opens and closes. Walter and I are alone – well, apart from Sweep.

'How are you feeling now, Walter?' I ask him, and he waggles his hand to indicate 'so-so'.

'You look quite tired,' I say, and he nods. 'Do you want to sleep?' I ask, but he shakes his head, saying, 'I have to fight this. The girls aren't ready. I have to keep going.'

'Walter, do you think it's not safe to sleep?' I ask.

Yes, he says. A liver specialist told him that in the end, he would die in his sleep.

'So, have you been fighting sleep for a while?' I ask, and he tells me that over the last few weeks he has needed daytime naps, and has found this very frightening.

'Walter,' *carefully, gently* . . . 'have you ever seen anyone die?' The question startles him, but he tells me that his father had a heart attack and died three days later, having been unconscious most of that time. 'Did he seem comfortable?' I ask, and after reflection, Walter says that his dad died 'in a good way'.

'What was good about it, Walter? What makes a good death, do you think?'

Walter says that his dad wasn't frightened, and that his family was around him. He woke up now and then, and smiled at them all. In the end, he just stopped breathing. 'We weren't really sure whether he was gone. I thought: that's the way to do it! But my heart is OK, so I won't die like that.'

The door opens and, firing me a warning glance, Walter immediately stops talking. Suit daughter, now in jeans and a T-shirt, brings a tray of steaming mugs into the room. PJ daughter and Molly join us, now more conventionally dressed. Walter asks for water, and Deidre shows the family how to help him to use a straw, expertly supporting his back so he can lean forward to sip safely. Then everyone grabs a mug, and the normalising power of a family sharing a tea break allows the next step of this drama to take place.

Between Walter's daughters in dining chairs at the head of his bed, and Molly sitting on it, I kneel beside Sweep again. Sweep patiently refolds his paws. Deidre leans against the kitchen door. We sip our mugs, and I open the discussion.

'Walter was just telling me about when his dad died. How peaceful it was, for his dad and for the family. He'd hoped it might happen like that for himself.'

There is utter silence. From beneath the bed, we hear Sweep scratching himself.

'Walter, you said you didn't think it would be like that for you, because you have a different illness from your dad. So you might be glad to know that what you saw is what dying usually looks like . . .'

Walter raises his eyebrows to indicate surprise, and I ask permission to share some information that may help everyone to feel less worried about what will happen to him. He looks anxiously at his daughters, and I promise that I will stop if anyone finds it too hard to hear. Walter gives a thumbs-up, then reaches out for Molly's hand.

I explain the 'gradually having less energy' phase, when a person's life expectancy is becoming shorter, and we discuss how this has been happening to Walter over the last few weeks. It was this change that made Walter's GP decide to discuss his priorities with him, and Walter had said that he wanted to be comfortable and peaceful, and not to be rushed into hospital for treatment. This was recorded in his Emergency Health Care Plan, so even if Molly had called an ambulance or an emergency GP who did not know Walter during the night, they would have avoided a hospital admission and managed his sickness at home, just as his GP and Deidre were doing now.

Reminding everyone not to let their drinks go cold, I move on to what to expect once a person who is weary enough to die no longer has the energy to get out of bed: the gradual increase in daytime sleeping, and the gradual reduction in time spent awake.

'From here on, Walter, I'm expecting only that you are going to feel more tired, and to need more sleep. I hope we can manage this sickness with the drug Dr Green gave you before she left. We'll put it into a little pump, and it will flow slowly into your body through a tiny needle under your skin. Deidre will be in charge of keeping it running well' – Deidre salutes Walter with her mug of coffee, and he smiles at her – 'and if the nausea comes back, then I'll come back too, to see what else we might need to add.'

'We'll try to avoid that, please, Walter,' quips Deidre, and everyone smiles. Despite Walter's fears, the atmosphere in the room is relaxed and cordial.

'So, at the very end of somebody's life, Walter, they're usually unconscious, not just asleep. That's what you saw with your dad, isn't it?' Walter nods his head thoughtfully, and I continue, 'And just as seeing your dad's peaceful death has comforted you, so you can do that for your lovely daughters. They will see what you saw: a peaceful dad, mainly asleep, sometimes awake, finally unconscious, and that very gentle change in breathing. Just like your dad.'

Molly surprises us all by saying, 'I've seen that happen. Just like you said. When my husband died. He'd had a terrible chest for years after working in the mines. We both knew it was coming. So I'm not frightened, Walter, and I'll be right here with you and the girls.' She turns to them and says, 'If that's all right with you?'

PJ daughter leans her tearful face towards Molly, and notices that Walter is holding her hand. 'Like Pauline said, Molly, you are family, and we really want you to be with us. Don't we, Dad?' Walter raises his hand, still holding Molly's, and gives another thumbs-up.

I ask if anyone has any questions, then join Deidre in the kitchen, where she has anticipated my plan and brought a syringe-driver from the car. Together we do the calculations. I write the prescription, Deidre draws up the drug, which we check together, then she clips the syringe into the pump, puts in fresh batteries, checks the indicator light, and we go back into the living room.

Walter is asleep with his mouth open. He looks even more waxy. Pauline is weeping quietly, and her sister is hugging Molly.

'Dad just told us that he loves us all,' reports Pauline, 'and he's sorry he never asked Molly to marry him.'

'Silly noddle,' sniffs Molly. 'I didn't need a ring. He's been my life. He knows it.'

The girl hugging Molly pats her arm and says, 'We know, Molly, and we know how happy you made him. We're so glad you're our almost stepmum.'

This love-in, as a family understands itself possibly for the first time, makes me look more closely at Walter. I cannot waken him. He has told his family how much he loves them; he has asked forgiveness for his regret; he has expressed his last wishes. And now he is deeply relaxed, and comatose. His breathing is slow and noisy. His skin is cool. His fingertips are blue. His circulation is shutting down, and when I feel for his pulse it is weak and thready.

'Walter?' I say loudly. He doesn't flicker in response. I open one of his eyelids, and an unseeing eye doesn't attempt to blink. Unconscious, and changing far faster than Deidre and I had anticipated. I catch Deidre's eye, and she frowns to show me that she too recognises that Walter is dying in front of us.

Inviting the girls to move their chairs closer, and finding another chair for Molly so that all three are gathered near the head of the bed, I kneel again and offer Walter's hand to Molly.

'Can you see how he's changing?' I ask softly.

Pauline says it's lovely to see him asleep so peacefully, but her sister looks from me to Walter to Deidre and gasps, 'Is it happening now?'

'I think it might be,' I reply gently, 'because his breathing is changing. Can you see how relaxed he is? No frowning now, not like earlier. Molly, what do you think?'

Molly lifts Walter's hand and says, 'Look how blue his fingernails are. I think it's time, and I think he knew. That's why he said those things.' This is a wise woman, and she has seen death before.

We don't want Walter's nausea to return, so Deidre sets up the

syringe-driver and tucks the little pump under Walter's pillow.
Then she has to leave for more house calls. As I am seeing her
out, she says, 'Well, I didn't see *that* coming.' I agree that it is a
sudden change, yet the signs were there over the last few weeks,
and Molly is not really surprised.

Back on the floor beside Sweep, I can feel my legs going stiff.
Every so often Walter takes a deep, snoring breath, and his
breathing becomes deep and fast for a while, then gradually slower
and quieter. I point this pattern out to the family. It is called
'Cheyne-Stokes' pattern breathing, and it signifies deep unconsciousness. Towards the end of each cycle of fast-to-slow breathing,
there are long gaps between Walter's breaths. I explain that eventually, during this very gentle phase of his breathing cycle, he will
simply breathe out, and then not take another breath. No panic,
no rush of pain, nothing spectacular. Only a gentle ending of the
cycle of breathing.

Sweep keeps putting his head out from under the bed and
gazing up at Walter, and at the faces around him. I can feel cramp
in my calf, and excuse myself to go to the kitchen and make the
next round of drinks, and to find some water for Sweep. I hadn't
intended to be here so long, but I know I cannot leave yet. I ring
my team to explain why I will be late back, and am just filling
the teapot when Pauline comes into the kitchen and says, 'I think
he's gone.'

And Walter has indeed stopped breathing. Still and yellow, he
lies on his bank of pillows with his head tilted towards his family,
still grasping Molly's hand in his. Molly is dry-eyed. Walter's
daughters hold each other and weep. Sweep is crying beneath the
bed.

'You have helped him to feel peaceful and safe,' I tell them,
'and he has died just the way he hoped to. You are a great team.'
Inviting the daughters to come closer, and to touch or kiss Walter
if they want to, Molly releases her hand from Walter's vacant grasp
and takes my hand instead. She walks me to the front window,

where she sits down and says, 'I can manage things from here. We'll be all right.' And I know that she will guide and support these two younger women as they say goodbye to their dad. The gift of witnessing a gentle dying has been passed to the next generation.

Stepping into the bright sunshine and the noise of playing children is shocking in its contrast to the quiet house. Life is going on all around us as this enormous event unfolds on the other side of the window. I call the GP to tell her what has taken place, leave a message for Deidre and the community palliative care team, and drive back to the hospital.

What a privilege, to be able to observe families as they are forged in a furnace of love and belonging, so often with its fiercest heat at the ebbing of a life.

Pause for Thought: Looking Beyond the Now

Stepping back to find perspective is a challenge. It requires the insight to acknowledge that there may be another way to look at a situation, and the humility to be prepared to examine our own view, and to change our mind if necessary. It may be easier to step back if we approach life with an attitude of curiosity rather than certainty, intrigued by what we may discover for and about ourselves. Sanjeev's young doctor was certain about what he needed; his nurse was wise enough to step back and see the bigger picture.

Stepping back is not easy, but it is always illuminating. In his essay 'My Own Life', written when he knew he was dying, the great medical writer Dr Oliver Sacks describes becoming able to see his life 'as from a great altitude, as a sort of landscape, with a deepening sense of the connection of all its parts'. He goes on to say that he feels 'a sudden clear focus and perspective'. This is the great gift that rewards stepping back – to look anew at what feels familiar and already thoroughly known.

The stories in this section of the book have included a variety of challenges to reinterpret a world that already seemed thoroughly known. Working with people whose minds may be confused, we can step back and hear their concerns, hopes and wishes expressed through the muddle. Working with people whose plight may seem unbearable to us, we can step back and find that their focus is still clear and worthwhile to them. Around a deathbed, we can see a group of people sensing, discovering and affirming the connection between them, or the feeling of kinship that is forged between strangers at a hospital or hospice, brought together in the shared and deeply emotional experiences at the end of life.

Because we will all die, many of us have developed a view about

whether or not we have a right to choose when to end our lives.
These views are based on diverse perspectives that include the right
to personal autonomy, the duty to protect the vulnerable, the
principle of equality before the law, the dignity of human life, the
fragility of the human condition, and personal beliefs based on
humanitarianism, on the great faiths, on utilitarianism, on virtue.
There is no doubt that campaigners on both sides of the debate
are motivated by compassion, conviction and principle. And yet,
the discussion is so often polarised, noisy and alarming, and seems
to bear little relation to what actually happens to people as they
approach the last stages of living.

Whatever your own view, it is likely to enrich your perspective
if you listen and carefully consider the opinion of those whose
view is different. Working in the reality of day-to-day dying, many
of us in palliative care roles are exasperated by the trenchant,
black-and-white opinions of the campaigners for either view, when
we know that the reality is neither white nor black, but a completely
individual, ever-shifting shade of grey for each person. The missing
perspective on both sides of the debate is the reality of human
dying, the unexpectedly gentle progression towards death that
most of us will experience, whatever the trials of the preceding
terminal illness.

Looking beyond the immediate situation offers us all a richer
perspective, and enables the dying to focus on what is most
important to them, whatever other ideas the rest of us might have.

Legacy

What a laden word. Legacy is what we leave behind in the world, for good or ill. It may be a deliberate and carefully curated collection of items; it may be the help or harm we have done as we interacted with others through our lifetime. The dying are often very aware of their legacy, and keen to ensure that their life ends in a way that does least harm to those they love. Some people work hard to provide memorabilia for others; some take altruistic action by fund-raising in the hope of relieving unknown others of the burden of disease; some wish to generate opportunities to create special 'last memories'. Whatever actions they may take with the deliberate intention of shaping their legacy, they may well be unaware of the multiple, nuanced effects that they have already had on other people's lives.

Something Unpredictable

Making a difference to the world seems to be an important life quest for many people, yet recognising the difference that we have made to the lives we have touched can be difficult for us. It is easy to dismiss our own contribution as insignificant, to compare ourselves with our peers and find ourselves wanting. Sometimes, the role of a psychotherapist is to help someone to re-evaluate their worth and their meaning, and to discover their true colours, shining through the humdrum of everyday life, and already appreciated by everyone except themselves. That in itself is a therapeutic win, and can transform a person's life.

And then, sometimes, fate just opens a gate that allows the unimaginable to happen.

'Be quiet! Dan's on the telly!' The family huddles towards the screen to watch a young man talking to a journalist on the news. Relaxed and smiling, he describes his interests: rock music, computer games, his dog. His expressive face, calm demeanour and articulate speech suggest he might be a young management trainee or a self-made businessman. The camera pans backwards; broad shoulders, like a sportsman's, come into view, and then as the shot pans out further, the appearance of his motionless body sitting in an electric wheelchair changes the context entirely. Dan is discussing death. His own death, likely to be in his twenties. His preparations for dying. And in particular his Emergency Health Care Plan, which will set out his carefully considered wishes if he is unable to express them himself in a medical emergency. Dan is campaigning for widespread uptake of Advance Care Planning.

The interviewer asks him to explain, and Dan outlines his

medical history. He was born with the gene that causes Duchenne Muscular Dystrophy (DMD), a condition that has been weakening his muscles since childhood. First he could play football with his friends, then he could only stand and watch, then he could only get there in a wheelchair, and now he controls his electric wheelchair with the small amount of movement he still has in his hands. He expected that during his twenties his chest muscles would weaken, his breathing become less effective, his consciousness gradually dim, and his life would ebb away.

But, by an additional twist of fate, Dan's DMD came with an extra complication: it has affected his heart, and could cause an unpredictable change in his heart rhythm that would result in sudden death. No warning. When Dan's heart condition was discovered, about eighteen months ago, he was offered an implanted defibrillator, a little electronic device to shock his heart back into action. Dan was poleaxed. He had accepted that he would die younger than his peers since he asked his mum when he was twelve, and she had the courage to answer him honestly. As his physical strength receded, he acclimatised to new ways of living in a steadily less able body, a body that would gradually take him to an early death. He got his brain around all that. But sudden death? At any moment, with no warning? That idea, quite understandably, boggled his mind.

My cognitive therapy service is for people whose minds have been boggled by their serious and life-threatening illness, and that is how I met Dan, a year before this TV interview. He was referred by a mental health team. They too had had their minds boggled by the idea of trying to help a suicidal youth regain the will to live while he carried on dying from two fatal diseases.

Flashback to our first meeting. Dan arrives at the hospice, where I hold the CBT clinic, with his parents. I watch him arrive, driving his wheelchair with confident ease, navigating corners and unfamiliar narrow doorways with languid skill. While I hold the door open, Dan manoeuvres into the therapy room and parks beside the desk. I offer the easy chair, but he can't be bothered with the lifting, hoisting and effort involved. We sit facing each other, and I ask him how he hopes I may be able to help.

He shrugs, and makes a multisyllabic noise that sounds like all the vowels of 'I dunno . . .' with matching facial expression – despair and challenge in one mooing word. He sits bolt upright in his impressive motorised chair, head bowed down. He is a tall, broad young man; with a different shuffle of his genes he might be a rugby player or a motorbiker. His red-blond hair curls at the neckline of his T-shirt. His perfect smooth skin, pale from living indoors, lies over muscles that no longer obey the commands from his brain. This condition only affects the muscles, so his sensation and thinking remain intact.

Although his mind is trapped in a body that is progressively resisting his will, I sense that Dan remains capable of imposing that will by the use of his intellect. I want to understand, and to help. This can only happen, though, if he agrees to communicate with me. But there was a challenge in that inarticulate verbalisation, and I am both professionally and maternally familiar with the ability of young adults to impose their will by withdrawal of cooperation. Only Dan can decide whether I am acceptable as a member of his team.

There is a silence. From his bowed-head position, Dan raises his eyes to look at my face. I gaze back. He looks down again.

'Dan, did you agree to come here, or were you just brought along?' I ask him.

He looks up, shrugs, and tells me that he agreed to come.

'So, can you tell me what you were expecting?'

He shrugs and makes the 'ayuo' noise again. I perceive that we are on thin ice. Is he going to let me in?

'You know Mr Purvis, who came to assess you at home, asked for this appointment for you?' I ask, and he nods, eyes averted.

'I think he wasn't sure how best to help . . .' I prompt him.

A slow, impish smile spreads over Dan's face. 'You mean I scared the pants off him?' he says. 'He just didn't know what to say to me.'

'Were you trying to scare him?'

'No. But it was funny listening to him trying to find a way to ask about things.'

I can imagine the poor psychiatric nurse being put through the wringer by the young man with two killer diseases and a suicidal depression. When is a suicidal idea simply an acceptance of reality? I can also see that Dan has a finely developed, dark sense of the ridiculous, and I recognise that this will be our meeting ground.

'So, Dan, you told him you want to be dead. How did he react?' I want to understand where the line is between being a person who accepts a life-threatening condition, and being suicidal.

Dan inclines his head sideways, fiddles with the joystick of his wheelchair, and tips himself back so that he is looking straight at me. 'Well, he kind of wanted me not to want to be dead, but he knew I had a terminal illness, so I think he didn't know what to say,' he offers.

I nod. 'And when you say you want to be dead, do you mean you want your illness to finish you off, or do you mean you want to finish yourself off sooner?'

His eyes open wide. He wasn't expecting such a direct approach.

'I don't know how I could do it,' he says. 'But I wish I could think of something.'

'Have you had any ideas?'

'I thought of driving my wheelchair into a lake. But how would I get there? And the chair would probably stop if the battery got wet . . .'

There is a silence. We share it. We are thinking, together, about Dan's predicament.

'No chance the battery would electrocute you first, I suppose?' I ask provocatively, and he smiles.

'Low voltage,' he responds. 'Health and safety . . .' A crackle of humour flashes between us; a creeping rapport has begun.

I observe his face as I ask my next question. He holds my gaze.

'Dan, what do you enjoy?'

Dan considers the question. He adjusts his sitting angle with his joystick. He furrows his brows as he thinks, then tells me that he used to love two particular computer games, in which he met his friends online and they competed or cooperated to solve quests. In one game he drove a car, in the other he had an avatar who could run, jump and fight – an able body, driven by Dan's mind. He enjoyed the questing, the thinking, the collaboration, and the online conversations he had with his friends. Time used to pass without dragging.

What was the best thing about it, I ask, and he can answer this without stopping to think. In his games he is the equal of his friends. He can compete, and he can win.

On the basis of my (limited) understanding of Grand Theft Auto, and our shared appreciation of the ridiculous, I am signed up by Dan for a trial on his team. He is articulate (when not in 'moo' mode) and smart; he quickly reaches an understanding that managing depression is a 'mind game', and he is very good at getting to grips with it. On days when his mood is lower, he is more inclined to shrug and moo. When I imitate his mooing, though, he heaves a sigh, then cracks a grin, and we game on.

We map his misery using a CBT formulation, and it looks like this:

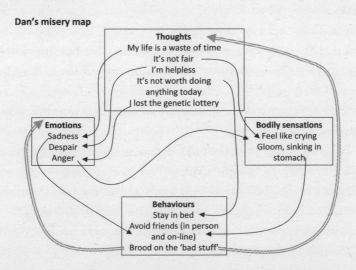

Dan's misery map

Over several weeks of regular CBT sessions, Dan and I discover lots of self-blaming thoughts that make him feel bad about himself. He believes he is a bad person, a selfish son, a critical brother, a poor friend. These are all common themes for people with depression. The depressed mind plays down positivity and eagerly embraces tiny examples of negativity, puffing them up into huge, undermining traps. It is like a malevolent spell cast by a mage in one of Dan's computer games; he needs a 'balanced mind' amulet, to restore his awareness of the hidden positives which are his protection against the Dragon of Despair.

He also resents the inheritance of a lethal gene, and the tipping point for his mood was the discovery of his additional heart problem. He has declined a defibrillator, causing some consternation in the cardiology team, but his logic is that a sudden death from an abnormal heart rhythm would prevent him waiting to die slowly. Why would a suicidally depressed person want to prevent their own death? His reasoning is faultless.

As part of his CBT, Dan experiments with activity levels at home and discovers that the more he does, the less unhappy he feels. This is the case for almost all depressed people. The challenge for Dan is to find ways of being busy when his voluntary movements are limited to minimal arm movement (he cannot lift the weight of his arms to scratch his own nose), movement of his neck and face, and enough hand movement to manage his electric wheelchair or Xbox controls. He rises to the challenge. Keeping a mood diary to log the effect of his efforts, he resumes internet gaming, he returns to his interest in rock music and even attends some gigs, he makes lists of his favourite music and then listens to it, he visits the cinema with his friend, he goes out for meals with his family, he notices when his mood is drifting downwards and gets busy, he pets his companion dog, and the family cat who sleeps all day in whichever room Dan is in; he even sings.

As Dan's mood lifts, we come back to the issue of control. He knows that his life expectancy is short – he is unlikely to see out his twenties, and the longer he lives, the weaker and more dependent he will become. He has phenomenal parental support: he lives as an autonomous adult in his adapted room where he controls the lighting, temperature and window blinds using his Xbox controller. He has help from his mum and a carer, a young man of his own age who has been a lifelong friend. His parents have managed to enable him to take risks that other families might not, like late nights out at a rock concert or cinema trips by wheelchair and public transport with pals.

For Dan, the loss of control comes if he is taken to hospital. Suddenly all the in-house knowledge of how to move him, hoist him, position him in bed, bathe him, is lost. Well-meaning staff either fail to listen to him or assume that his lack of movement is associated with brain damage, making him incapable of expressing his preferences. He hates hospital. He fears hospital-isation. He dreads being hooked up to a ventilator during a medical crisis, to find that he is then condemned to live with a ventilator when without it his natural death might have occurred peacefully. As long as he can remain at home, living as well as he can, and supported through any crises, he is content. What he cannot bear is the thought of an ambulance crew or hospital team that arrives on the scene during a crisis, intervenes, and prevents his natural dying. So, having succeeded in restoring Dan's will to live, we must now plan how to manage his death well.

Dying quickly from a cardiac arrest would prevent hospital admis-sion, so Dan still declines a defibrillator. He declares this 'not suicidal, just self-preservation'. There's a crazy logic that his family accepts. He also asks for a Do Not Attempt Cardio-Pulmonary Resuscitation order, so no one will resuscitate him by mistake. These are brave and delicate conversations, and Dan thinks through the options carefully. His magnificent parents, who want him to live for as long as possible and would take the defibrillator, a ventilator, a whole intensive care unit into their home if possible, support his decisions. Such empowering parental courage, such enabling of autonomy. This really is love in action.

The next piece of work we do is to prepare an Emergency Health Care Plan. In it, we describe Dan's medical condition, his understanding of his condition, and his preferences for levels of intervention should decisions need to be made in a medical emergency. We state clearly that if he is so sick that he will probably die, he does not want to go to hospital, but wants all care to be aimed at comfort and delivered at home. We describe his wish to be as awake and alert as possible, so that he can communicate, but also that if he is feeling very afraid or has severe symptoms, he would prioritise having symptoms managed over alertness. We express his carefully considered wish not to have cardiac resuscitation should his heart stop, as we know it might. We state his desire to avoid the use of a ventilator. And his wish that, if he has a medical emergency that appears reversible with hospital treatment, he should be admitted to hospital for treatment, provided he is discharged home as soon as possible; and if the hospital team cannot save his life, then he wants to come home to die.

Dan's many specialist medical and nursing advisers support us in writing this plan. His cardiologist reviews the suggestions for palliation of heart failure at home; the consultant from the home ventilation team wins Dan's confidence and tests his breathing capacity, showing that respiratory failure is not yet on the horizon, and advises about best management of future chest infections; the muscular dystrophy team comment on drafts. In working together on the document, we are distilling a vast amount of expertise into a carefully crafted plan that promotes Dan's wishes.

This takes several weeks, and by the end of it Dan has a complete protocol for what actions family, GP, district nurse, ambulance crew, out-of-hours emergency services and hospital emergency departments should take under specific circumstances, including a plan for end-of-life care at home with a box of 'just in case' drugs for use by community staff. This is all backed up by a DNACPR order. Dan, who now loves being alive, has a complete plan for how his dying will be managed. He finally, really, feels in control.

One of Dan's bleakest thoughts during his depression was that 'It was a waste of time me being alive. I won't achieve anything. I will leave no legacy.' Of course, part of his legacy was firmly in place: the enormous love and devotion within his family. Dan will be present forever for them. But his peers are making their way in the world, and the contrast between his life and theirs becomes ever more stark. While I was mulling this over, fate gave us a wonderful opportunity.

Dan's EHCP and DNACPR order were two of the forms involved in a region-wide collaboration to plan complex care in advance, respecting the informed wishes of patients no matter where their care takes place. By carrying his plan with him, Dan had a right to the same care whether he took ill at home or was scooped up by emergency services while out at the cinema, across a huge area of England. This was a national first (although sensible Scotland already had a national DNACPR order), and the regional NHS team had arranged a media launch of the documents. The intention was to raise public awareness and attempt to get people with serious illnesses to begin discussions with their GPs, hospital specialists and, of course, their families. As regional lead I was to write newspaper articles and be interviewed on radio and TV. But wouldn't it be so much more interesting and compelling if not I, but an articulate patient, could be interviewed? . . . Dan didn't need to be invited twice.

Fast forward to the launch date. Dan's mum generously opened her home to the media for a day. Dan was filmed, photographed, tape recorded. The journalists were utterly entranced by his down-to-earth discussion of his illness and his quiet acceptance of his early death. He explained his treatment plan and decision against resuscitation; he described the empowerment of having been able to discuss his condition openly and plan his future options in detail. He was broadcast on the radio and on two TV channels, and appeared in the newspapers. He was a Facebook and Twitter sensation. Within two weeks the numbers of enquiries on the regional NHS website jumped tenfold. Dan's clear, level-headed and generous sharing of the making of his end-of-life plans changed many more minds and melted many more hearts than anything I could have said.

But best of all, the consultant from the DMD team rang me to let me know that other young men with the same diagnosis as Dan had contacted the clinic to ask if they too could have 'those papers like Dan's'.

Unpredictable, yet absolutely right. Dan had the time of his life, and helped a whole community to consider putting more thought into discussing and planning their end-of-life care.

Dan's time and mode of death remain something unpredictable. The conversations that he was empowered to have by taking up advance care planning helped him to be better understood by the DMD team, the cardiology team, his own family, even himself – something that people often avoid, but that in the end is right. We should all have those conversations with our dear ones, and sooner rather than later. Thanks, Dan.

The Year of the Cat

The timing of each death is a mystery. Although we can anticipate when time is getting short, and indeed it becomes easier to estimate life expectancy as the end of life approaches, on occasion the moment of death seems to be related to something more than just the underlying illness. People we expected to die days ago wait until an important piece of news is announced, such as a birth or other significant event; people who have been continuously accompanied by family members somehow stop breathing during the only few minutes they have been left unattended; people who were expected to live a little longer find that a personal issue has been resolved, and relax into dying earlier than expected.

It's the community review meeting. The specialist nurses of the community palliative care team are discussing the new patients they have seen this week, usually at the request of a GP or district nurse. These specialists, often referred to as 'Macmillan nurses', have additional training and expertise in palliative care and will help the primary care team to manage most patients' physical, emotional and spiritual distress in their own homes. For particularly difficult-to-manage symptoms, admission to the hospice might be requested. It is the early days of the in-patient hospice, and the Macmillan nurses have their office here, so as a young trainee I am able to attend the review meetings, and sometimes I am entrusted with deputising for our leader. Today is such an occasion.

The next patient is introduced by Marian, a livewire with a vibrant sense of humour and wonderfully Home Counties delivery. She presents the story of Bob, an elderly recluse living in a council flat in a run-down suburb of the city. Bob has advanced cancer in his mouth and neck. He is a proud man who declines help, and Marian had to conduct her first discussion with him through his letterbox. She produces a collection of pages roughly torn from a notepad. Bob's cancer started in his tongue, which makes his speech almost unintelligible, and as Marian boomed her plummy questions from one side of the door, he had issued his replies on paper through the letterbox. Towards the end of their interview Bob had opened the door to let his cat out, and the stench of stale food, stale cat and stale human had almost overwhelmed Marian. She chose to admire the cat; Bob invited her in.

She found Bob smartly dressed in grubby clothes: checked shirt; trousers so loose that he needed a belt; a waistcoat and cravat. His swollen lips and cheeks were red from wiping the drooling saliva that poured from his irritated mouth. He led the way into a living room piled high with boxes and plastic bags, filled with – what? Marian spotted a bag full of egg-timers, another full of old news-papers. Some boxes held rubbish, whilst others clearly contained carefully collected items. Some bags simply held dozens of paper tissues daubed with drooled saliva. Only one chair was visible amongst the debris: an ancient, upholstered armchair made shiny by years of use that had ingrained and polished the grime. Bob gestured to indicate that Marian should take it, and she coura-geously perched herself on the very edge while Bob threaded his way through his grotto of belongings to the kitchen, returning with two cups of tea in British Rail mugs. He sought his pad, and wrote:

Unfortunately I am unable to offer milk.

Bob brought in a kitchen stepping stool and sat at Marian's feet, constantly dabbing away his saliva with tissues while conversing using his writing pad. He was frustrated when saliva dribbled onto the paper, and would rip the page away and begin writing again in order to present clean pages, a process that doubled his writing time. From this conversation, Marian understood that Bob had constant pain in his mouth and one cheek, that he was becoming less and less able to swallow his painkillers, and that his cat was the centre of his world.

Bob's cat had been chased into his flat by a local dog about a year earlier. At that time it had looked around six months old. Bob had just completed radiotherapy to his mouth and was very tired, often too tired to shop, cook or eat. The arrival of the kitten changed his order of priorities: he got up every morning to let it out; he walked to the supermarket to buy cat food (indulging his new pet's fastidious taste for the most expensive food available); he retrieved a blanket from amongst his collection of bags and folded it into a pet bed. Financial necessity meant that the fussy cat received only meagre portions of food, so it spent all day rubbing itself around Bob's legs and purring, to be rewarded with a tiny allocation of cat biscuits. Bob had never been so loved, nor felt such companionship.

The problems Marian brought to the community review meeting were Bob's pain, and Bob's cat. Bob needed a period of in-patient care to manage his awful pain, but he was unwilling to accept this because he had no family, friends or neighbours to whom he could entrust the care of his bewhiskered next of kin. Marian herself was a cat-lover, and perhaps that was partly why Bob had trusted her to come into his flat. Her own cats would not tolerate Bob's kitten as a visitor, but she could lend me anything I might need to take in a little kitty-witty for a couple of weeks while we just . . . *Wait! Me? I don't like cats!* I have been scarred, physically and mentally, by an early catty acquaintance. *No way!*

Marian's eyes filled with tears. 'He's a little tabby with white paws. He's small for his age because Bob can't afford much cat

food. And he's got the sweetest face . . .' She holds her fingers
beside her cheeks, like whiskers. 'You'd love him!'

Marian doesn't understand 'no'.

That evening, I try to choose the best moment to announce to
my husband that we are taking a physically retarded tabby cat on
a two-week foster placement. As anticipated, the news goes down
badly. Unlike me, my husband loves cats, and grew up with a
series of them. It would be cruel to lock a cat in our house while
we're at work all day, he protests. What were you thinking? The
answer is definitely no.

The cat is delivered by Marian in person before we leave for
work the next morning. She hands the cat-carrier to my husband,
who, despite being an Immovable Object, can recognise an
Irresistible Force when he meets one. Game over.

Bob has a bed in a four-bedded bay, and Marian says he looks
'splendid' after a luxurious bath (he declined any nursing help).
He is given a pair of pyjamas, and he accepts because all his own
are contaminated by saliva (and grime). He agrees to allow the
hospice housekeeper to launder them for him. Marian alone is
entrusted with a key to Bob's flat. He asks her to bring in his
clothes, and also all his cat treats to give to me towards the cat's
bed and board. Marian brings Bob's clothes two days later, in one
of her own suitcases; Bob is delighted to note that they are much
cleaner and better pressed than he had remembered . . . Marian,
with her heart of gold, is wondering how to help with his flat
next.

At home, the domestic rhythm of our mornings is changed at
a stroke. The beast eats a massive breakfast in the kitchen, then
runs amok for thirty minutes before I can capture it and manoeuvre
it into Marian's cat-carrier. It chooses a different place in the house
to anoint with its smelly urine every day, and we play 'hunt the
cat poo' every evening, led by pungent clues. No wonder Bob's
flat was whiffy.

I deliver the cat to Bob each morning. It tours the four-bedded bay with its tail erect, sniffs the corners of the room, then jumps onto Bob's bed and curls up to sleep behind his pillows, purring gently.

Bob was a perfect patient. He was courteous and appreciative. It took time to converse with him thanks to the combination of his fastidiousness about the state of his paper and the slow concentration with which he carefully formed each letter of his copperplate calligraphy. He was willing to experiment with painkillers delivered by injection, so that he would have no need to swallow tablets. As his pain improved he began to walk around the hospice (cat on arm, syringe-pump in pocket), but he quickly became tired. He pined for his flat and his own personal space, and so, two weeks after he arrived, he was ready to go home. Time for me to talk with Bob, to plan his discharge from the hospice.

I was sitting beside him when the cat jumped onto my knee and settled down, purring. *He has developed a fondness for you*, Bob wrote on his pad. I couldn't help feeling absurdly pleased; the purring transmitted a trembling warmth all over my body. *You have provided an affectionate lodging for him*, wrote Bob.

I smiled. 'It's been our pleasure,' I said, and in that moment I realised that I meant it. The cat had taken to a litter tray (husband's experienced intervention), and the loudness of his milk-associated purring was remarkable. He had doubled the household milk order single-pawedly.

He should remain domiciled with you now, Bob ominously penned on his pad.

Uh-oh!

'Bob, whenever you need a break, then the cat can come back to us. But he's your cat. We can't take him away. He is your family,' I said. 'Besides, my husband will think I've talked you into it.'

Bob wiped his mouth. I noticed there was bloody ooze in his

saliva. *Show this to your husband,* he wrote, *as evidence of my intentions and of your innocence.* He carefully tore a clean page from his pad. With fastidious precision, he wrote the date on the top of the sheet, and then inscribed in his careful, artistic hand:

I am glad that the cat
will be yours for ever
and ever.
Amen.

And then he signed it with enormous care,

Robert Oswaldson.

That evening at home, the cat was discussed again. We were DINKys – Dual Income, No Kids. We were out all day, and were both on call many evenings and weekends. We were sitting exams and writing up theses and really, really, didn't need a cat.

We took the unusual step of visiting Bob in the hospice together. He was a bit sleepy, but acknowledged our presence by sending me to make tea for all three of us. And milk for the cat. We repeated that we would offer foster care whenever needed, and Bob nodded, stroking the purring cat. It was Bob who extracted a promise from Immovable Object that *after the Inevitable* his cat would become ours. Bob was satisfied with this Gentlemen's Agreement.

On call that Sunday evening, I got a call from the hospice. Bob was restless, pacing the room and shouting, although his speech was so distorted that no one knew what he wanted. He was too agitated to use his pen and pad. He had tried to throw a chair at one of the nurses. Earlier, his pulse had been rapid and his temperature raised, but now he would not let the nurses re-check. 'Please come and assess him.'

It took less than five minutes to drive there. Bob was standing in the middle of the room, wearing only pyjama trousers. His frame was wasted and tiny, but in his disturbed state he was very strong. The nurses had removed the other patients to the calm safety of the TV lounge. I went in and sat with a nurse beside Bob's bed, where the cat was curled up behind the pillows, indifferently washing its paws.

'Bob, come and sit with us,' I said, then ducked as a teacup was hurled across the room. I pulled the cat out onto the counterpane. 'Come and stroke him,' I suggested, 'because it's nearly time for me to take him home.' Bob stomped across the room and picked up the cat-carrier, initially swinging it like a weapon and then placing it on the bed, at which (to my astonishment) the cat immediately jumped in and lay down. Bob began to tie the door closed, and as he bent down I could see bloody saliva dribbling through a hole that had appeared in his cheek. The skin of his cheek was crimson, and so swollen that the pores looked like craters pitting a shiny, smooth, red lunar surface.

'Bob, your cheek looks very sore. . .' I began. He looked up, catching my eye directly, and shook his fist. Was he angry with us? With his pain? With his situation? He sat heavily onto the bed and began to cry, sobbing and rocking and wailing, possibly trying to speak, yet utterly unintelligible. I touched the back of his hand, but he shook me off, roughly shoved the cat-carrier at me, and pointed to the door. The message to take the cat away was clear.

The nurse and I went into the corridor with the cat. From there we could keep an eye on Bob's safety without inflaming his wrath any further. The combination of new, red swelling up the side of his face with high temperature, fast heart rate and agitation all suggested a bacterial infection in the swollen, juicy tissues of Bob's face. This is a recognised complication of head and neck cancers, and is usually associated with severe pain. The fever can cause confusion, and it was this that was causing him to become agitated.

From the corridor I could see that the redness was already extending to his ear and down his neck. The pain would be horrible. He needed antibiotics in high doses, by injection, and clearly I could not treat him while he was fighting us all. If I could give him a gentle sedative he would feel calmer and less agitated, and then I could get a needle into a vein and treat his infection, his fever and his escalating pain. But he was unable to swallow. How could I help him?

As I was pondering that thought, Bob suddenly and unexpectedly got into his bed, and within minutes was deeply asleep. The nurse and I approached. His cheek was swelling visibly and a second new hole was dripping saliva. He stirred when we touched his arm, but did not withdraw or open his eyes. I tried to ask his permission to give an injection; he pulled his arm away.

'I think he wants us to stop,' said the nurse. 'He's had enough.' It seemed that she was right. I called the leader, and he came in to assess the situation. By now, Bob had developed twitching of his limbs, and irregular breathing. The leader considered several possible reasons why Bob might be twitching, and feared that he might be at risk of having convulsions. Yet again we came up against the problem of how to give him any medication that would stop his twitches and prevent them becoming fits. The rectal route seemed the only way.

The rectum has such a rich blood supply that drugs given by this route take effect very quickly. In France, it is a usual way of administering medication even at home. In England, however, we use this very effective route less regularly. I wasn't sure that Bob would understand that we were trying to help, but asking his consent was not a possibility while he was so muddled and afraid. With heavy hearts, a nurse and I prepared the smallest syringe that could deliver the dose of a drug that would prevent fits and also offer some sedation.

Two nurses and the leader helped to hold Bob in a position that would allow me to place my blunt syringe as gently as possible into his rectum and squirt the drug in. It felt intrusive as he wriggled and shouted. I was weeping as I said, 'I'm so sorry, Bob. This will really help you. That's all we want.' And then it was done. Within five minutes the twitching stopped; five minutes later a peaceful Bob was deeply asleep, and a small injection port was taped into a vein in his arm. No need for any further rectal drugs, with a venous route established. I took the cat home.

The injection port was a vital part of Bob's care for the next few days. Over that time he remained mainly asleep, waking occasionally to give the cat a biscuit and stroke his purring body. The antibiotics reduced the redness, and Bob's pain and temperature settled, but he did not improve. That lack of energy we had already observed was, as usual, a reliable indication that Bob's battery was running low. He had managed the single most important matter in the world – the future care of his cat. With that resolved, he was ready to relax.

Bob died three days after his troubled weekend, without getting home, the cat on the bed beside him.

The final chapter of Bob's story provided a little illumination. With no (human) next of kin, Bob had no one to register his death or arrange his funeral, and the hospice took on those tasks. I made my first ever visit to the local registrar's office to deliver the medical certificate of death usually taken by the family. In a room populated by an incongruous mixture of beaming new dads and the silent newly bereaved, I handed in my certificate and explained the unusual circumstances to the clerk. Then I sat and waited.

Eventually the chief registrar bounced out of her office and greeted me like an old friend. 'Ah, Dr Mannix, what a pleasure to meet you at last! We've followed your career with interest!' That early run of fourteen deaths in ten days jumped accusingly into my mind. Then my time at the cancer centre. And then at a hospice. Goodness me, they must have typed my name a lot of times over the years. It had never occurred to me that this could be a way of monitoring a medical career – this was many years before a registrar of deaths was to sound the alarm over the now notorious GP and mass murderer Harold Shipman.

'Sorry about your wait,' she went on, 'but we had to check the rules, because we've never encountered a situation where a death was registered by the same person who signed the certificate. But it appears we can proceed.' She produced the official copy of Bob's death certificate, and the form I needed that allows an undertaker to dispose of a body by cremation or burial.

The mourning party was small when we assembled at the cemetery: Marian, the hospice manager, and me as a representative of Bob's cat. There we encountered a distant cousin of Bob's, and an erstwhile colleague from his days as an employee of the railways, who had seen the death announcement in the local newspaper. We stood together in the cemetery chapel while a minister who knew neither Bob nor his mourners made an attempt to comfort us in our loss, and then we watched as Bob's coffin was lowered into the earth.

Walking away from the grave, Bob's ex-colleague said, 'I didn't know he had a daughter.' I explained that I wasn't Bob's daughter, I was his – friend. 'I'm glad he had friends,' the man said. 'He was a lonely type of guy. Kept himself to himself. It's a responsible job, being a signalman. He used to worry. Deep thinker. Kept meticulous records, and always beautifully written. He was a lovely writer.' Almost as an afterthought, he added, 'And such a curious turn of phrase. He talked like an old book. Old-fashioned. Loved his long words . . .'

He tipped his hat and walked away, leaving me to consider Bob's life, now reduced to a pad of prosaic communications using poetic language, all expressed in copperplate calligraphy.

Then I went home to feed our cat.

Post-Mortem

The examination of a body after death may be to establish why a person died. This can help in unexpected deaths, but is rarely a question in palliative care. Yet sometimes, even though the decline and progression towards dying is understood, there are questions unanswered after the death, and an autopsy examination can help to address these.

Of course, the patient is beyond benefit from these post-mortem answers, and that fact raises the question: what is the point? I believe the point is that our mutual interconnectedness, our belonging to each other, enables these too-late-to-help answers to be of use to other people: to offer a deeper understanding of how an illness was affecting the person as death approached; to answer questions about the impact of previous treatments like surgery or radiotherapy; to give new insights into causes of symptoms that were hard to manage. It is not idle curiosity: autopsy offers answers that can benefit future patients, progress research, and comfort the bereaved. But if we fear discussing death, how can we ask permission for this last, definitive exploration of a person's dead body and the impact their illness had?

Besides, what colour is cancer?

Moira is furious. She flushes pink and balls her hands into fists. She stares at me, as we sit in the hospice staff room, then almost spills her coffee as she stands and shouts at me.

'How can you? I mean, really – how *can* you? Hasn't she suffered enough? I cannae believe you want to do that . . . that . . . awful thing!' And then, to her frustration, her anger turns to tears and she sits down suddenly, searching her nursing uniform pockets for a tissue. The rest of the team cast their eyes downwards, apart from Sister, who is looking at me, then at Moira, then back to me, to see how this will play out.

'Moira, tell me what's so awful about this for you,' I say.

Moira flushes again. 'We're here to care for her. It's bad enough that we never got rid of that horrible pain for her. But to cut her open now she's dead – what good is that going to do her? And to ask her family. They'll be even more upset than they already are. I just didnae expect this of you. No, I didnae! I'm appalled . . .' She trails off, lip wobbling and eyes brimming.

Our patient Ruby died last night. It was an expected death: she had widely spread cancer, and had been semi-conscious for the last three days. She had been in the hospice for three weeks, and over that time we had reduced her distress, enabling her to be comfortable enough to sit in a wheelchair and be taken around the gardens by her family, and to discuss her funeral arrangements with her son. But we had never made much difference to the most upsetting pain, an odd circle of discomfort sitting just below her navel and slightly to one side, that caused her to cry, rub, wince and shriek without warning. We had tried so many things: heat (hurt), ice (hurt), drugs (no help, even at doses that made her sleepy), nerve stimulator (really hurt), hypnotherapy (brief reduction), distraction (interrupted by shrieks), massage (intolerable to be touched there).

I was a new consultant. This team of nurses, a social worker, physiotherapist and occupational therapist had worked together for years, and trusted each other. Adding consultants to this established hospice was a new venture, and I was still on probation. It had seemed to be going so well. We were nine months in, and now, suddenly – this.

We had all found caring for Ruby a challenge. Her pain did not fit any textbook patterns – it seemed to come on whenever she felt other patients in her room were getting more attention than she was, and it was always more shriek-inducing when her family was visiting, causing them to demand that we 'do something', as if we were not trying.

'I'm not sure that a bereaved family can be more bereaved,' I say. 'We all feel frustrated that we never got on top of that odd pain, and I want to know if we missed something. I know it won't help her, but it would help us, and it might help the family to have an explanation. And it's knowledge we can use for other patients. That's why I want to ask.'

'How can they say no?' demands Moira. 'I mean, if it's going to upset them, but the consultant asks them, then how can they say no?'

I hadn't previously thought about the power balance in these conversations, but Moira is making a valid point. I have not yet got used to the altered status that comes with the title 'consultant'.

'Would you like to come with me, and act as an advocate for the family?' I ask. Then a new possibility strikes me. 'In fact, of all of us, you know them best. How would you like to offer them a chance to find out more about that pain, and if they agree, then I'll come to explain the procedure and get consent signed?'

Moira looks astonished, but Sister says, 'Great idea. They really trust you, Moira, and they could say no to you, couldn't they?'

Later that morning, when the family arrive for Ruby's belongings, death certificate and our condolences, a nervous Moira goes to meet them in the lounge. After ten minutes or so she reappears on the ward and says, 'Well, I'm astonished, but they *would* like to ask more about a post-mortem. Can ye come up?' I love Moira for her integrity. She could simply have followed her feelings and ducked the difficult question.

In the bright and airy lounge, the family is gathered in an alcove around a low coffee table, where traditional tea-and-sympathy is being served. I kneel beside the sofa, at the feet of Ruby's son and daughter-in-law, and ask what they would like to know. Moira sits on the arm of the sofa.

'A post-mortem . . .' says her son. 'It's kind of like cutting her open, is it?'

'Yes, that's right. It's a way of having a really good look at why she had that horrible pain that we never really got rid of for her. It will show us things that a scan can't always see. The part of her that I really want to know more about is the inside layer of her tummy, under where that pain was, and all the nerve supply to that area. A full post-mortem looks at the whole body – inside the tummy, inside the chest, and inside the head. But we can ask for a limited look around, if that's what you prefer.'

The family agree that they would want Ruby's head left alone, and I assure them that this is fine. They want to know where the operation will happen, and when.

'The procedure would be done at our local hospital, by experts. So you can visit her here today, and after that you can still visit her, but over there. They'll do it today or tomorrow, so that it won't hold up your funeral arrangements. And I'll go, maybe with Moira or another member of the team, to see exactly what they find.' Moira's eyebrows arch with surprise – I hadn't mentioned that in our previous discussion.

Acknowledging that this procedure is of no help to Ruby, and that our whole team feels sorry that we never got rid of her pain, I explain to the family that if the autopsy helps us all to understand what was causing it, it will help us to help other people. And every cancer post-mortem helps the doctors to understand cancer a bit better.

'But – and this is really important,' I stress, '– I can give you a cause-of-death certificate today. I don't need a post-mortem for that. So if you think the idea of a post-mortem is going to upset you, it's really fine not to go ahead.' Moira nods at me approvingly.

'No, we've decided it's a good idea,' says Ruby's son. 'We'll always wonder. And Mum always brought us up to help people, so she would like the idea of carrying on helping now. It's fine. We'd like to go ahead.'

I produce the consent form, and explain about how Ruby will be handled. There will be a single, long cut to take out her organs. They will be carefully examined, and small samples may be removed to be looked at in more detail through a microscope. That extra process may take many days, so all but those small samples will be put back inside Ruby, and she will be carefully stitched up again. The family won't see cuts or stitches if they visit her later in the hospital's chapel of rest, and the funeral can go ahead as planned.

Ruby's son signs the form. I tell the family that I'll be happy to see them again to discuss what the examination shows. It's best to wait until all the information is back, including any microscope work, so we should plan to meet up in several weeks' time. I ask them to phone us when they feel ready. Then I issue the cause-of-death certificate, and return to the ward while Moira explains to the family how and where to register the death.

Later, we are all gathered in the office once more. Moira has something to say.

'I didnae mean to sound disrespectful when I shouted at you earlier,' she begins, her Scots brogue highlighting her discomfort. 'A nurse shouldnae speak to a doctor like that . . .'

I feel deeply touched, yet anxious, to hear these words from such an experienced and wise colleague. If we are a team, then we must feel safe to disagree with each other. No doctor should ignore the advocacy of nursing colleagues. Nurses spend far more time with patients and families, and every team member's view should be offered with the confidence that it will be listened to with respect. Am I really part of this team yet?

'Moira, please don't ever think that nurses can't hold doctors to account – that would be so wrong!' I say.

She flushes. Then she smiles at me. 'And what's this about going to watch?' she asks. But the anger has left her voice, her anxiety about overstepping has passed.

'Well, we want to know, don't we? So we'll go and watch. Would you like to come?'

'I'm not sure . . .' she replies, so I say that I'll phone the pathology department, get a time for us to go across, and if she wants to come, she will be welcome.

Leaving to attend the post-mortem later that day, I call into the ward to see which of the nursing team, if any, are willing and able to attend. I find Moira and Sister with their coats on, looking apprehensive but determined. They are on a mission to assure themselves that their patient remains cared for with dignity in the hospital mortuary. We arrange to meet in the car park in five minutes. This gives me just enough time to rush into the secretaries' office, call the mortuary manager, and warn him that I am bringing two nurses to their first ever autopsy. I have known Keith for years; he reassures me that 'Everything will be hunky-dory, as usual.' Then I collect my colleagues and drive us all across to the hospital.

Because my husband is a pathologist, I am on first-name terms with the whole mortuary team, each one of whom has a heart of gold and a genuine desire to manage these last days of their clients' visible existence with dignity and respect. In their care are the bodies of the very old and the newly born; the once sick, the fatally injured, the murdered; the loved and the unloved – the dead of our city. They treat each body with tenderness: indeed, Keith has taken it upon himself to find a way to use invisible glue to seal the post-mortem wounds of the babies, so their families can cuddle them without feeling stitches through their tiny pyjamas. Tina chats to every corpse as she conducts them to the giant refrigerated shelves in which they will repose. Amy makes sure that no child's body is ever left alone, a promise she makes to keening mums as they tear themselves away from the viewing-room cot. This is the Kingdom of the Dead, and it is a place of dedicated kindness. I know my colleagues will not find fault in here.

Keith meets us at the back door of the mortuary, a route known only to undertakers and staff working in the Kingdom. He welcomes Moira and Sister, and tells them that Ruby and Dr Sykes are expecting us. He asks us to put on plastic overshoes and operating gowns, and I suddenly realise that, rather than taking us into the viewing gallery, from where we could watch through glass (no smell), we are being taken into the autopsy room itself. *Not what I was expecting.* I brace myself for the nurses' reaction when they see the four dissection tables with naked bodies being eviscerated and examined.

Silly me. Keith opens the door to reveal that each table bears a body covered by a sheet, only the head and toes visible. Ruby is closest to us, and Keith asks the nurses to walk around and join him beside Dr Sykes. Facing them across the sheet that covers Ruby, I see that Sister is pale and Moira radiant pink. Dr Sykes is clad like a surgeon in all respects except that rather than clogs he is wearing big white rubber boots. I notice a covered tray on the draining board of the sink beside him, which I know holds the organs he has removed from Ruby's body. *We don't have to watch the dissection; what a relief.*

Dr Sykes explains to us that he has already completed the first part of the post-mortem. Ruby's body has been opened, and he was able to see lots of cancer deposits as he looked at her lungs, her liver and her guts. He beckons the nurses over to the draining board with the covered tray. I steel myself for their shock. He peels back the cover, to reveal a smorgasbord of purple and grey meat: liver, lungs, heart, intestines, kidneys. I see Sister rock back and reach for her handkerchief, but Moira moves to get a closer look. Dr Sykes points out the place in Ruby's intestine where her original colon cancer had been removed and the ends rejoined – the tiny, glistening pearls of cancer studded along the shining surface, filling the lymph nodes; the cancer-ball projecting out of her liver, which he opens deftly with a long knife, dividing the liver into parallel slices and spreading them like a fan to show glistening white cancer deposits from golf-ball to pinhead size; the blizzard of tiny cancer seedlings throughout her lungs.

Moira's rapt attention is total. 'White!' she exclaims. 'I never expected it would be white. I just imagined it would be red, or black – an evil colour. I've been looking after people with cancer inside them my whole career, and I never knew what it looked like . . .' She stares intently, shaking her head in awe.

Dr Sykes says he has found cancer deposits in Ruby's spine, and I wonder aloud if this might account for the odd abdominal pain. He offers to show us the spine.

'Where is it?' asks Moira, still closely examining the contents of the tray.

'Still inside her,' replies Dr Sykes, moving to lift the sheet. Keith steps forward to help, and deftly folds back the sheet to the level of Ruby's waist. Sister looks away, but Moira cranes her neck for a better view. We are looking inside Ruby's ribcage.

'Hello, Ruby,' I say. 'I've brought Sister and Moira to see what was causing all the bother.'

Dr Sykes points to the spine, which looks like a line of children's building blocks running down the centre of Ruby's body cavity. One of the blocks is misshapen, and from it there glistens an odd protrusion, like a crystal in a rock: a cancer deposit. It is at the wrong level to account for her abdominal pain, but it explains why she had pain in her back.

Dr Sykes asks for more detail about the abdominal pain, then begins to run his gloved fingers slowly along the insides of Ruby's lower ribs. He stops and says 'Aha!' then invites us to put on a glove and feel in the same place. Beneath the eleventh rib on the right is a tiny lump, impalpable from the outside. The bottom of each rib forms a tiny protective gutter along which runs the slender, vulnerable nerve that transmits sensation from that segment of the body. In this particular nerve, in this tiny space beneath Ruby's rib, there is a cancer deposit the size of a grain of barley. It is in exactly the right place to 'scramble' nerve messages from the segment of her trunk running from just below her umbilicus, diagonally up her abdomen, under the rib and around her back to the spine. This tiny, unsuspected deposit of cancer was responsible for Ruby's pain. Nerve pain is always hard to describe, hard to bear, and often difficult to treat. Soft touch (like massage) or nerve stimulators in this segment would increase the sensory messages and the painful scrambling – just as we had seen in Ruby's last weeks of life. We have our answer. Thanks, Dr Sykes. Thanks, Ruby's family. Thanks, Moira.

In the car on our way back to the hospice, Moira is ecstatic. 'I cannae believe cancer is white!' she says. 'And who would ha'e thought there would be that tiny lump on her nerve like that? No wonder we couldnae stop her pain!' There is no advocate like a convert, and the successful identification of an unsuspected cause of pain had converted Moira entirely to the value of post-mortem examination. 'I'm so glad we have something tae tell her family,' she says. 'And we'll always wonder whether weird pains might be nerve damage from now on – I just know this will help us to help more patients. That was just . . . well . . . it was incredible. I'm so glad I came to see.' I am so grateful that the mortuary team has managed our visit with such sensitivity, and that Moira has such an open-minded passion for nursing.

That was only the first of our post-mortem adventures. Moira's advocacy ensured that all our nurses were aware of the value of finding out after death what had confounded our attempts at symptom control during life; she encouraged every nurse to attend a post-mortem if they could. Not all had such a Damascene conversion as hers, but all found it a help in understanding the illness that confronted them on a daily basis.

These days, Moira is a senior nurse tutor in a university school of nursing. Her students are all encouraged to attend at least one post-mortem.

Needles and Pins

Legacy is a complex concept. Is our legacy a tangible object? Is it the memories of us that other people reflect on? Is it the difference we have made in other people's lives? And how can a teenager create a legacy? Well, here's one who did. This story is another piece of it.

Sylvie is nineteen. She is a drummer in a band. She was planning a career in music management, something to do with sound mixing and the technical manipulation of recorded sound. She likes loud music with a pounding rhythm, but she also writes haunting ballads with gentle, lilting melodies that remind her of being rocked to sleep as a child. She is an only child, a precious treasure to older parents who delighted in her birth, celebrated every milestone of her life, and are now preparing themselves for her imminent death.

Sylvie has a rare type of leukaemia. She had gruelling treatment with chemotherapy for her sixteenth year of life ('So missed out on GCSEs and alcohol. But still managed drugs and rock'n'roll,' she smiles). After another year of trying to rebuild her stamina enough for her to return to school, her leukaemia relapsed, and this time treatment is not winning. Despite this, she is possibly the most smiley person I have ever met, made even more so by her dazzlingly white teeth ('I'm the missing Osmond sister!' – smile) and her startlingly vivid choice of lipstick, contrasting with the snowy pallor of her face, and by the ever-so-slightly-sideways tilt of her Cleopatra-style black wig. ('Oops! Adjusting headpiece!' – smile.)

Sylvie's leukaemia-producing white blood cells crowd everything else out of her bone marrow. The drugs that are applying a diminishingly effective brake on the leukaemic cells also damp down other, useful cells. This toxic combination of rampaging white cells and suppressive drugs reduces the production of red blood cells, making her anaemic (pale, lacking in energy, easily breathless), and of the tiny blood-cell fragments called platelets, that ensure cuts and bruises clot off quickly. Sylvie is surviving because other people give blood; she has a blood transfusion every week, and she needs transfusions of platelets on alternate days. Her survival is dependent on the kindness of strangers.

This dependence on dripped-in blood products would usually mean that she had to live in hospital, because blood products can cause allergic reactions or fluid overload, so patients are monitored constantly during transfusions. Sylvie considers herself 'lucky' (smile) because although she is now legally an adult, she has a childhood-type leukaemia, and is still under the care of the region's children's cancer service. This provides nurses who will deliver transfusions at home if absolutely necessary, and when you are down to your last few months of life (smile), well, that's a time you want to spend at home, isn't it? (Smile.)

I am on a training placement with the children's cancer service as part of my 'knit your own' training in palliative medicine. This includes being embedded in the team of children's cancer specialist nurses. These inspiring nurses work with newly diagnosed children and their families to support them through whatever combinations of surgery, chemotherapy and radiotherapy they require to manage their cancers. They visit GPs and community children's nurses to brief them on the support and care the child may need at home, because most GPs will only deal with one or two children with cancer in a whole practice lifetime. They visit schools to advise teaching and pastoral care staff on how to support classmates, and how to keep in touch with the absent pupil, because most teachers will never teach a child with cancer.

The odds of being cured of cancers arising in childhood are

much better than for adults, and the cancer team goes all out for cure whenever possible. But, of course, some children relapse, and others don't get into remission in the first place. Then these nurses offer a palliative care service aimed at keeping life as normal as possible for as long as possible. They visit the children at home, and advise parents on nutrition, exercise, school attendance, symptom management, and how to discuss the illness and its implications both with the patient and with other family members, including brothers and sisters. They advise the GP and community children's nurses about palliative and end-of-life care, because most GPs will not have experienced this before. And they support teachers who are, in turn, supporting a class of children who are anticipating, and then mourning, the death of one of their class-mates. What a job.

I don't have most of the experience needed for this role. I am not a nurse, I have no experience of working with children (my only relevant child-health qualification at this point is rearing my three-year-old son), and only some of my adult cancer experience applies to the treatments these young people are having. I am clinically qualified, though, and Sylvie is technically an adult, so she is assigned to my caseload, and I have come to her house to meet her, along with the nurse who knows her best.

It is late autumn. The house is in a remote village, along twisting lanes. I am observing the route closely, because next time I come I will be on my own. I will be responsible for bringing the platelet transfusion bag and a drip set, to administer Sylvie's transfusion and to monitor her while it runs. The low morning sun is catching the frosty leaves in the hedgerows, fringing them with golden haloes. The glory of the autumnal display sits uneasily with the purpose of our journey. How on earth will I know what to say to this dying teenager and her parents?

The house is yellow stone, standing alone amongst tall trees at the edge of the village. The wooden, farm-style gate is open and a gravel drive curves around mature bushes. There is a cattle grid

at the gate, and it jangles loudly as the car crosses it into the drive.
By the time we park and collect bags and boxes from the car boot,
the front door is opened by a smiling woman holding a tea-towel,
and through the open door the sound of drums reverberates into
the morning air. Our breath is visible as we scrunch across the
gravel. The drumming stops, and a window opens at roof level.
A bald head wearing headphones pops out and declares, 'You look
like dragons!' before the window slams shut again and the lady
in the doorway welcomes us inside.

The nurse introduces me to Sylvie's mum. Sylvie's mum gestures
around the huge farmhouse kitchen, warmed by a squat, ancient
Aga-type stove, and apologises for 'the mess'. The mess seems to
be an open newspaper and a teacup lying on the table. Or perhaps
she thinks we can see her soul.

A door opens cautiously and a gentle voice asks, 'Where's
Friday?'

Mum replies, 'In his cage,' and I notice a golden retriever sitting
very quietly in the corner.

Sylvie, no longer bald, slides in around the door, and Friday
gives a cheerful bark. She walks gently, carefully, as though she is
walking on ice. 'Hiya, team!' she greets us, beams at me and gives
the nurse a hug, before draping herself carefully into the corner
of the sofa, where she folds in her long legs, tucks her lopsided
hair behind her ears, nods at the dog and says, 'He knocked me
over yesterday. I'm as wobbly as a skittle!' (Smile.)

I recognise this picture. Some chemotherapy drugs damage
people's nerves, dulling their ability to feel their fingers and toes
while cruelly replacing normal sensation with pins and needles
– some people feel as though they are walking on shattered glass.
This makes it difficult to walk with confidence, and people do, as
Sylvie says, become wobbly as skittles.

The nurse asks about bruises: Sylvie's low platelets increase the
spread of any bruise. Sylvie smiles – the radiance of that smile is
like a lighthouse on a dark night – and says ruefully, 'Yep. Landed

on my bum. Looks like I'm growing a tail.' She turns sideways, pulls down her loose leggings and shows us the dark purple bruise that spreads across her left buttock and down her inner left thigh. 'Ouch!' says the nurse, and Friday whines softly. 'You didn't mean it, silly pup!' comforts Sylvie.

Over the next hour I discover that Sylvie is astonishing. Her mum stays for the first fifteen minutes, and then withdraws – 'Thanks, Mum. See ya later!' (smile) – giving Sylvie a chance to talk without worrying about upsetting her. As soon as she leaves the room, Sylvie fishes out a bag from beneath the sofa and produces its contents – some coloured fabric, baby clothes, T-shirts, a piece of thick foam and some sewing materials. 'It's going to be great!' she tells the nurse, and between them they introduce me to the Project.

Sylvie got the idea while she was in hospital a couple of months ago. A play therapist was helping two youngsters to make clay models from a kit. One was picking her model (she chose Mrs Tiggywinkle) and putting clay into a mould, the other was painting the model he had made previously (Percy the Small Engine). The children were excited – these were 'surprise presents' for their parents. 'But you didn't have to be an Einstein to see how sick those kids were,' Sylvie said. 'And then I watched them make handprints in the clay. That's when I realised that they were making presents for their parents to remember them by. Kind of goodbye gifts . . .'

Sylvie thought about this for a while, and came up with the Project. She shows us the fabrics. 'I'm trying to choose all Mum's favourites. This bit is from one of my old sun dresses. That's one of my baby vests. And this is from a T-shirt I painted at Guide camp when I was twelve. That button is from my school uniform, because I was always losing buttons and she kept having to sew on new ones' (smile). The foam will become a round cushion, and Sylvie is making a patchwork cushion-cover from her own clothes – from her mum's memories.

Sylvie's mum only takes a break from her daily chores when she rests in front of the warmth of the kitchen stove each evening. She sits on a battered rocking chair that was once her mother's, and that should have been a legacy to Sylvie. This memory-cushion is for the family chair: an enrichment of the legacy, for a future that Sylvie will not see.

There is a rustling outside the door; the bag is whisked away. Mum brings in a tray of steaming mugs of coffee, then turns to leave us. 'You can stay, Mumsie,' says Sylvie. 'There's no Big Stuff today.'

After coffee and taking a blood sample, the nurse and I say goodbye. We explain that tomorrow's platelet run will be done by me, while the nurse goes to deal with a child at the other side of the county who has just started chemo. 'Poor chap,' says Sylvie. 'I hope he wins.'

The next morning, I start my day at the haematology lab. I know all the technicians from previous work in adult haematology, so I drop in to say hello. They remember me as a rookie – my very first post as a doctor. I collect Sylvie's blood-test result (platelet count eighteen, normal range 200–400) from the lab, and am then escorted next door to the transfusion lab to collect the platelet bag for her.

'Look out! She's back!' they joke. They ask what I'm doing these days, then ask, 'And how's Sylvie?' with earnest interest. Although they spend their working lives in the labs, these kind people have followed her story, and those of others like her, through the medium of blood counts in and blood bags out. They recognise this pattern of failing treatment. They know that she is dying, that soon the blood tests will cease, that she will not see out her teens.

'Cheerful and creative,' I say, 'and looking forward to your excellently prepared platelets, which I shall serve with coffee and a biscuit.' They pass me the padded, insulated blood-products bag, like a small lunchbox, and I set off.

'Give her our love!' shouts the chief lab technician. He has probably never met Sylvie, but he has been in the lab since very early this morning to defrost her platelet transfusion so it can be given early in her day. What a service.

Today it's grey; no golden light or dainty frost. The county is shrouded in fog, and none of the roads look familiar. I am very relieved to drive across that cattle grid and up the noisy gravel. I gather my kit: blood bag (check); notes and observation sheets (check); rucksack with novel in case patient wishes to snooze through transfusion (check); medical bag with drip set, stethoscope, thermometer and blood-pressure cuff (check). The front door opens, Friday runs out to sniff me with huge enthusiasm, and Sylvie is in the doorway, wigless, smiling (of course) and saying, 'You should see my bruises!' in welcome.

Sylvie's mum takes the opportunity of a two-hour medical visit to get out to the local town to shop. She shows me where to find cups, coffee, milk, the telephone. Sylvie's dad is at work; the dog will be happy to wander around the garden. It's just the two of us. We begin the platelets ceremony: check temperature, pulse, blood pressure; run the drip through using saline; take sterile dressing off Sylvie's special intravenous line; connect saline drip, check it runs smoothly; swap saline bag for platelets; note the time; observations every fifteen minutes.

'So, there's a big problem,' announces Sylvie. She looks downcast. I ask what she means.

'With the Project. Stupid fingers are numb. I can't sew. I can't feel the needle. I can't hold the fabric straight. Stupid. Stupid, stupid, stupid.' She bites her lip.

'Poop,' I agree. She looks a bit startled. 'Medical jargon,' I assure her.

'Yeah, right.'

'What's the plan then?' I ask.

Silly question: *I* am the plan. Within seconds she has produced the workbag, scissors, pins, a tape measure. Sitting with me at the huge kitchen table, she directs while I pin and sew small squares of fabric together. She surveys, changes, tilts her head sideways while she considers, sucks in her cheeks, shakes her head, moves fabric squares. Intermittently our attention is diverted into the observations of pulse, blood pressure, temperature, and then we are back on task.

While we work she chats about her family, her music, her friends, being bald, body image, legacy. Legacy is such an unusual word for a teenager to use, yet she really means it. Her school has run fund-raising events for leukaemia research, mainly concerts to which Sylvie has contributed either in person as a drummer, or remotely by editing tapes that were sold at the events. These tapes will be in circulation after she is dead, and she finds the idea fascinating, compelling, sad yet consoling. Being bald is 'a nuisance in the winter, brrrr!', but on the other hand, 'It's quite a cool look for a girl on stage.' Her body-image issue is 'hamster cheeks' induced by steroids. Her changed facial appearance continues to startle her – 'I share the bathroom mirror with a girl I don't know.'

She moves back to legacy. 'There's two parts to that. There's living on in my music, and that's kinda easy to get. Like, other people have already done that, haven't they? John Lennon, John Bonham, Keith Moon . . . They made that noise in real time, and it's like they're here now when I play those tracks. But the other bit of legacy's harder. It's so sad for Mum and Dad. Dad has his work, he stays busy. He's keeping it out of his head. I'm quite like him, really – I use drumming to stay sane. Mum, though, she's different. She'll be tough, but it will be so hard for her, being on her own while Dad stays busy. We sit here by the stove in the evenings, Mum and I. Just snuggle down, a chair each, a cup of tea. Just chatting, or thinking. That's when she'll miss me most, I reckon.

'That's what made me think of a cushion for her rocking chair. It's my way of saying, when I'm not here any more, "Come and sit on my knee, Mum." And I can rock her, and she can feel my arms around her, as we rock together in front of the stove. It's genius. I hope she'll like it.' I cannot look at her, and the sewing is becoming blurred. I concentrate on not dripping tears onto the fabric. *These tears I gotta hide . . . needles and pins . . .*

By the end of the transfusion the patchwork is assembled under her direction, and I have stabbed my own fingers multiple times. Pins and needles spike my fingertips as I gather my bags; they have less in them than when I arrived, but somehow they feel heavier. They are filled with admiration and awe for this almost-woman, this great-hearted human, who has lived and loved so fully in a lifetime cut short, whose cup is half full – no, in fact, so full it is running over.

Lullaby

Offering a palliative care service to strangers is an intellectually stimulating challenge, filled with job satisfaction. It's very different to be walking a palliative care route alongside our own dear friends and family, especially when the disease is stripping away the delights of childhood from a much-loved baby. This story is about the wonderful resilience of families in the most heartbreaking of circumstances, and a legacy that preserves a beloved child's name as a word associated with comfort and care.

It's hard to believe what I'm hearing my friend say. The evening light is skimming the hedges outside the lounge window and shafting into my eyes as I stand beside the telephone. I am blinded by the brightness, and all my focus is on the words she is saying in a calm voice – deliberate, carefully rehearsed phrases, cautious care in her words, measuring her ability to communicate such dreadful news.

'Do you understand what I'm saying?' Lil keeps repeating, and I realise that I am failing to communicate the horror that is creeping through me.

She is a paediatrician. She understands baby and child development, and she notices tiny details the rest of us might not. Now on maternity leave with her gorgeous twin girls, she has been relishing watching them change and develop, step by step; interpreting their gurgles and chuckles, delighting in their pleasure as they discover their fingers, their toes, their voices; and sharing, within our little friendship triad, the joy of becoming a mum and of learning the ropes of parenthood with her husband.

But she noticed a tiny detail that I certainly would not have seen. One of the twins, Helena, had developed very fine muscular twitching in her tongue. In a bright, happy and beloved baby, this was a shocking sign to her knowledgeable mum: a muscle disease that is progressive, debilitating and fatal. By the time my friend was ready to tell us her terrible news, Helena's diagnosis had been confirmed by a specialist. Spinal muscular atrophy (SMA), Type 1 – the most rapidly progressive form of all. Helena was unlikely to reach her second birthday.

'Do you understand what this means?' Lil asks again, and I am nodding – not helpful on the phone – because I am utterly lost for words. This is cruel, and dreadful, and these are twins: a horrible thought shoots into my awareness just as she is saying, 'We're so thankful that they're non-identical. Saskia doesn't have the gene.' I cannot fathom how they can be thankful for anything at all as they ponder what lies ahead.

We have been friends since medical school, Lil, Jane and me. Lil specialises in child protection, which sounds unbelievably sad and traumatic to me. She will find it harder now she is a mum. Jane is a children's anaesthetist: she manages tiny people through huge operations, and often works alongside colleagues in a children's intensive care unit, another unspeakably difficult and stressful job. Yet they think my choice to work in palliative care is equally challenging. So between the three of us, Jane points out to me on the phone when we talk the next day, we have all the knowledge that will be required for Helena's best supportive care for her short lifetime. How ironic.

Jane is looking ahead. She knows the progress of SMA from her work in intensive care. As the child's throat muscles fail, they become unable to swallow safely or to clear phlegm from their airway, so their lungs are prone to infection. This is compounded by progressive weakness of the muscles in their chest, so they cannot cough or take deep breaths. Simple colds can become overwhelming chest infections. Early on in the condition, admission to intensive care and temporary use of a ventilator to support their breathing enables them to return to live at home, while their muscle failure slowly progresses to reverse the milestones of rolling, sitting, crawling and standing that they have so proudly achieved. Further on in the condition, the child may be incapable of more than the slightest movement. Fed by a tube for safety, and requiring constant attention to remove saliva that they cannot swallow from their mouths, yet fully mentally aware and attached to their families, there may come a time when admission to ICU is simply prolonging dying rather than restoring health. They may no longer have the muscle strength to breathe without the ventilator. Many families cannot manage a ventilator at home, and the child is tethered to life by a ventilator and to hospital by the need for ventilator management. Jane has seen families unable to recognise when promoting living has segued into a purgatorial extension of dying without hope of improvement. She is horizon-scanning for problems – that's why she is good at her job.

My small contribution is regular telephone conversations, using my CBT knowledge to help Lil separate out her realistic, sad thoughts about the future from catastrophic imaginings that turn every day into a minefield. Out and about with both girls in their twin buggy, she is used to a mixture of admiring glances and inane or intrusive questions like 'Are they twins?' 'So they're the same age, then?' 'Did you have IVF?' Now, these same villagers appear to her to be avoiding her, crossing the road as she approaches or hurrying away towards bus stop or car park. Her world is suddenly full of twin buggies – mums and grannies with healthy twins, normal life expectancy, 'just taking it for granted' and fuelling her bitter anger and despair. Much of this is simply her own reinterpretation of events. Helena doesn't look unwell, and as yet there is no reason for any passer-by to suspect that there is anything out of the ordinary about the threesome as Lil strolls around the shops with the buggy or attends nursery singing with the girls. Unhappiness grows like a weed that takes root in imperceptible cracks in our psyche. Lil and I examine her experiences, identify the weeds, and she vigilantly uproots them as she feels her mood slipping.

The presence of a healthy twin means that some kind of balanced family life must go on. While they are small enough, each twin sits in a backpack when their parents take them on wilderness walks in the Pennines or their beloved Scotland. Initially at least, both achieve their motor milestones, Helena sometimes a little later than her sister, but within the bounds of normal development. Both love music, both love bathtime, both love each other. Like many twins, they can be content in each other's company for long periods of time, chuckling at a shared joke or admiring each other's hand movements, mesmerised by such a companionable soulmate. They 'talk' to each other for hours: Lil phones us so we can listen in and marvel at these deeply meaningful, utterly unintelligible conversations.

Helena's first serious chest infection arises suddenly, and she is in hospital, in an isolation room with oxygen to support her breathing, very quickly. Her parents take turns to stay with her while the other tries to keep life as normal as possible for her sister. And yet, for Saskia, how can life be normal without Helena? Jane stays in closest touch over this period, her anaesthetist's brain vigilant for signs that ventilation may be necessary, and Lil finds her contact comforting. I manage a flying visit, chatting to Helena through the transparent tent that maintains a higher oxygen level for her breathing, and joining Lil in a nursery-rhymes medley. Helena is panting and her ribs shiver with the effort, but she still manages to laugh at us. Priceless. She gets home a week later without the need for a ventilator. This time.

Aged two, the twins are beautiful and aware of it, reeling me in with smiles, and responding with a clear 'No!' to most maternal instructions. Ah, I smile to myself, the terrible twos have arrived. While the instruction-resistant behaviour is to be expected, what is unexpected is that both twins are still here. As if to illustrate their evolving disparity, Saskia runs across the room to where Helena lies on the sofa; she clambers onto the sofa (nice mantelshelf manoeuvre – you can tell her parents are mountaineers) and launches herself over the back, while Helena lies motionless apart from her eyes, which follow every move of her agile and entertaining sister.

Helena can now only continue to breathe because other people observe her constantly, ready to suck strands of mucus and dribbles of saliva from the back of her throat where they pool, gurglingly obstructing the flow of air in and out of her lungs. This can mean using a little suction device thirty times an hour; deeper suction with a miniature vacuum cleaner is needed at less frequent intervals. She tolerates this intrusion, which she has no power to resist, with remarkable equanimity, occasionally furrowing her eyebrows and flaring her nostrils in protest, but smiling again as the tube is withdrawn from her mouth or nose.

The exuberant development of new skills and tricks by one twin mirrors her sister's inexorable decline. The depth of Helena's loss is illustrated by Saskia's motor agility and emerging speech. And yet, Helena smiles and gazes, and enquires, and flirts, using every piece of her might to be part of the quadrangle of love between twins and parents. Her parents contemplate the expected death of this indefatigable daughter, and wonder at her daring and strength to have so outlived all expectations, every day a precious, fragile burden. Sleepless and exhausted, carried by willpower and dread of her distress, how much longer can they dare to hope to have her? How much longer can they bear to hope? I watch my weary, courageous friend with awe, while Helena bathes her family in the grace of her happy presence for a little while longer.

The phone rings around lunchtime while I am writing teaching materials at home. It is Lil. Is she crying? My heart lurches. No, she is laughing. She can barely speak. 'I'm calling on behalf of Heli, who has something important to tell you. Here she is . . .'

I can hear noisy breaths. Helena's facial weakness makes her
speech hard to decipher, but what I hear is 'Ka? Ka?'

It's my name. 'Hello, Heli, here I am.'

'Ka! Monna nor-ee tep!' Giggle. Fast breathing. Giggle. Lil
provides translation – *I'm on the naughty step.*

'Goodness! On the naughty step! What have you been up to?'
I ask, intrigued that she is capable of such wickedness, and delighted
at her delight at her own mischief.

'Ontid orter!' (*Wanted water*) she trills merrily.

I can hear Lil laughing, then she says, 'No, don't look at me,
I'm only here to hold you. This is the naughty step. No chatting
with Mummy for two whole minutes!' Heli giggles again.

'Kath, this little lady is supposed to be having her nap while
Saskia is asleep and Mummy does some work. But she wants to
play with water and bubbles. She keeps shouting from the sofa
across to me. And she has been asked to wait. She has been warned
to give Mummy ten minutes' peace. She has been warned that
one more shout and she will have to sit on the naughty step. So
here she is!' I hear the sound of the saliva sucker in use, along
with more toddler chuckling.

Heli comes back on the line. 'Nor-ee tep!' she splutters. 'Like
Ash-ya!' *Naughty step! Like Saskia!*

'Yes, Saskia is a regular attender here,' laughs Lil. 'But this is
Heli's first ever time, and she's so pleased with herself.'

Two hilarious minutes are up, and Lil carries Helena back to the
sofa to bask in her triumph. I assume the phone is tucked under
Lil's chin; no wonder she is getting a bad back. She sucks more
saliva out of Heli's mouth while telling me how wide Heli's eyes
are with smiling – now more indicative than her mouth. We say
goodbye for now. As Lil rings off, I hear Heli demanding, 'Orter.'

My dear friend. Keeping it 'normal'. Disciplining her daughter,
because that's what normal looks like. The love between them
almost palpable as they share this precious moment. I am so
delighted that they shared it with me.

The family were active in seeking advice to help Helena to remain as well as possible. They were disappointed to discover that, although palliative care services for children with cancer were fairly well developed, there was almost no provision for children with other lethal diseases. Lil's ruthless exclusion from the house of anyone with a cough, a cold or a sneezing child protected Helena from chest infections, and by networking, online research and sheer determination, she and her husband found specialists to help reduce Helena's symptoms. They visited a clinic in Scotland, where Botox injections into her salivary glands reduced Helena's saliva, drooling and need for suction; they found physiotherapy experts who advised them about optimising her muscle function and keeping her chest clear; they assembled a trusted team to sit and watch over her whenever they could not be present, enabling some snatched hours of sleep at night knowing that her saliva would be suctioned and her posture changed regularly to keep her comfortable. Her survival now demanded constant supervision to ensure saliva did not block her airway.

The twins enjoyed three birthdays together. This was a stunning survival time for a child with Type 1 SMA. They spent family holidays in Scotland, went hill walking, and Helena's chairs and bed were adapted to enable her to sit and participate as fully as possible in family life. Helena focused her keen intelligence on a laptop computer (a novelty at that time), and used it to create colourful computer-generated animations to accompany her favourite music.

Although Helena's horizons were shrinking, her three-year-old quality of life was lovingly maintained by her family, who had helped her to outlive her original two-year prognosis and who continued to find inventive ways to enhance her life. When Saskia began to attend nursery, coming home with new stories about friends unknown to Helena, Lil was able to have one-to-one time with Heli so that she too would have news to tell Saskia when they were reunited. The girls were bridesmaids at their cousin's wedding, clad in 'princess dresses' and very pleased with themselves, Helena in her chair and Saskia firmly on guard beside her. They were particularly proud of their silk ballet slippers: Saskia's were quickly worn ragged, while her sister's remained poignantly pristine.

Jane was very much afraid that Helena's next chest infection would only be survivable by using a ventilator, and that her chest function was now too poor to escape the ventilator afterwards. She expressed concern that Lil and her husband would find it too hard to turn down the chance to extend Helena's days by any means. But not knowing how to broach this discussion, we simply waited and wondered, marvelling at Helena's life of utter bodily stillness and intense mental activity.

And then Helena became hot and breathless. The diagnosis of a chest infection was apparent to her mum immediately, and a decision needed to be made. Heli loved being at home, surrounded by her family and her familiar team, her own bedroom and her beloved toys, and she disliked the noise and unfamiliarity of hospital. So it was decided that she would stay at home, with fans and cool sponging, drugs to relieve breathlessness, extra oxygen as needed, and no ventilation. This meant that she could be cuddled by the family, and feel them close. She was unlikely to survive, but her parents' love and forethought, as in all the other aspects of her short life, had prepared them for this decision.

We need not have worried. As Heli became drowsier and less aware, Lil rang Jane. Jane rang me. We wept and we waited.

On a bright June day, sitting with her family and while 'Walking in the Air' played on repeat, Helena became very drowsy, her shallow breathing developed long pauses, and then stopped. She was entirely surrounded by her dearest people, and there she remained until her funeral, dressed in her 'princess dress' and ballet slippers, on a special cooling mattress in her bed, and surrounded by candles and flowers.

What a wonderful funeral. The undertaker delivered a tiny white pine chest to serve as her coffin, and her parents snuggled her into it from her bed only immediately before the service began. We gathered in the living room. Heli was brought downstairs to the dining table, resplendent with candles and flowers, and the local vicar conducted a service of thanksgiving and farewell. Then the chief mourners loaded up their camper van and set off for Scotland, where Helena was to be buried in a plot purchased some time ago for that purpose.

They broke their journey at Jane's home overnight, then continued to the rugged beauty of the Scottish wilderness to commit their redoubtable daughter to the majesty of the craggy and familiar landscape.

I learned from this experience how families develop their under-standing of the meaning of an illness over time. When the diagnosis was first made, this devoted family would have stopped at nothing to keep their daughter alive for as long as possible. And yet, quietly and lovingly, over time their position shifted. They purchased a grave site, they focused on tiny details that yielded enormous benefits to their girls, they recognised the diminishing odds of adding quality to life, and they bowed with grace and tender dignity to the inevitable, ensuring that Helena's death was as enhanced by love as the whole of the rest of her life.

They also determined to ensure that other families dealing with SMA should have better access to condition-specific palliative care. They fund-raised, often by walking (and requiring friends to walk) huge distances in Heli's beloved wilderness, and they established the Helena Nursing Team of specialist nurses supporting SMA patients and their families.

When I asked Lil for permission to tell their story here, many years after these events, she was eager that I should record this fact: in the hospital canteen queue that very day at work, the person in front of her was a nurse specialist whose badge said 'Helena Team'. She didn't know who Lil was, she may not even have known who Helena was – but evidence of her legacy filled Lil's heart.

Pause for Thought: Legacy

What legacies have you already inherited from people now dead or no longer known to you? Perhaps material things like books, ornaments, money. Perhaps mementos like letters, postcards, or their modern electronic equivalents. Possibly stories handed down through your family. Maybe you were encouraged as a child by a particular person, or modelled yourself on people whose qualities you admired. These are all forms of legacy.

What legacy have you already generated? You may have given birth to children or to innovative ideas; you may have taught a grandchild how to use a screwdriver or how to see pictures in the clouds; you may have founded a major company or grown a garden. You may have borne sorrow with courage that inspired other people, or quietly supported another in their time of need.

What legacy would you like to leave? Perhaps you are an organ donor; perhaps you have gifted a legacy to an endeavour you wish to support in your will; perhaps you are already preparing memory boxes or albums for your loved ones.

By modelling a way of dealing with a truth that society tries to hide, you can begin a legacy that calls death by name, accepts that it is a part of life, and encourages others to do likewise.

Who would you like to support in becoming less fearful about dying? How might you engage them in talking about wishes and preferences in later life or as death approaches? How might you help each other in this task?

Transcendence

The human mind applies itself to many more tasks than simple survival. We are aware of our personhood, and we seek to create a personal meaning from the jumble of our life experiences. Most people adopt some kind of framework that allows them to recognise and respond to the values that give them a sense of purpose. For some their framework is religion, or politics; for others it is the cycles of nature, or the vast unfolding of the universe. For some it is a more immediate system of interpersonal relationships, or thoughtful appreciation of music, art or poetry. Whatever the framework, this search for 'meaning beyond and yet including myself' is a metaphysical construct that is the spiritual dimension of being human.

In an increasingly secular United Kingdom, we struggle to find words and concepts to discuss spirituality without recourse to the traditional language of religion. Whilst members of faith groups may derive enormous benefit and comfort from the traditions and rites of their religion, sometimes these same traditions cause problems that may be difficult to identify and attend to for carers who do not share their beliefs. This is likely to be an increasing challenge as we become both more multicultural and more secular.

Yet at the end of life, many people make a 'spiritual reckoning' of their worth and the meaning of the life that is ebbing; they seek to transcend the difficulties that beset them, and to consider a bigger picture. This impulse allows extraordinary acts of courage and devotion, of humility and compassion, supported and validated by their personal spiritual constructs. It is perhaps that spiritual dimension of humanness that reveals us at our very best, even (or perhaps especially) here at the edge of life.

Musical Differences

There is a period of most lives in which we are dying. Sometimes
we are aware of this as we live through it, and sometimes it is only
apparent to the bereaved in retrospect. Yet the important label of
this part of life is 'living' rather than 'dying'. Even at this end time,
the discovery of new things, making new friends, learning and
growing are all still possible, still fulfilling, still worthwhile.

In adjacent rooms yet unknown to each other, two individuals
look back with satisfaction and forward with uncertainty. Different
diseases have brought them here, to their edge, and different
ideologies inform their views of it. And yet so similar; so similar,
like a recurring motif in a symphony.

They share a love of music. His is classical: he is a connoisseur
of Mahler, and now he finds his beloved music too poignant to
listen to. Hers is jazz: she once sang like Billie Holliday. They
share a healthcare background. He is a retired eminent psychiatrist
(I regularly find myself bumping into retired presidents of medical
royal colleges who visit him), and she is a retired hospital cleaner.
They both have wonderful, entertaining tales of hapless incidents
in the lives of the great and the good, to which we hospice staff
listen with a mixture of mirth, disbelief and schadenfreude.

He was admitted to our hospice with a huge and inoperable
abdominal tumour. He had spent his life in medicine, treating
teenagers with psychological distress and training medical students.
Indeed, at a critical stage in my student career he had helped to
persuade me not to abandon my studies. Now he was troubled
by pain from his tumour and anxiety about the strong medications

that might be needed to control it. A career working with the young had afforded him little experience of the dying.

On arrival he was examined by one of our junior doctors. She reported that he was playing down his pain and trying to 'maintain dignity'. He believed that confusion, drowsiness and indignity would rapidly follow any attempt to use morphine for his pain. She had tried hard to convince him otherwise, but he was adamant. His first priority was to maintain his intellect so that he could continue to support his family emotionally, and he was prepared to accept any pain to achieve that. 'He retired before I was born,' my trainee said ruefully. 'Doesn't he realise things have moved on since then?'

Startled by this declaration (*Surely I was a student far more recently than that?*), my 'How can time play such tricks?' calculator abruptly informed me that I was old enough to be my trainee's mother. So when she told me that she reckoned we would have to bring in the Big Guns to challenge his misapprehensions about morphine, I realised with a sinking heart that she meant me, the 'boss' who, until thirty seconds ago, had simply seen us as fellow women in medicine, sisters in arms.

Under the circumstances, I waited until after he was settled into his room before going in to introduce myself. Despite being a Big Gun, I didn't feel I needed or wanted the full consultant ward-round gun carriage present for our discussion of life, the universe and morphine.

Twinkle-eyed and sandy-haired, he was still recognisable as the kindly, powerful presence I recalled from my student days, but now much diminished, folded up like a deckchair as he perched on his bed with his back against his pillows and his knees pulled up towards his chest, a full fold-up prevented by the massive lump protruding from his lower abdomen. He was pleased to know that I had once been his student, and that I felt it was a privilege to take my turn now to serve him. He couldn't possibly remember every student, and he had the grace and integrity to grin and inform me that since he didn't recognise me, I must have been well-behaved.

I asked him to describe his cancer journey so far, to let me understand what troubled him most and what his priorities were for his time at the hospice. His GP had asked for him to be admitted because of the severity of his abdominal pain and his reluctance to try any of the medications offered to him at home. With a rueful grin he said, 'I'd better introduce you to Bruce.'

Bruce, it turned out, was his tumour – so named because 'he came from down under'. Bruce was initially removed by a surgeon, but returned and grew in size and vigour over the next few months, wrapping himself around several vital organs and blood vessels, thus assuring himself and his host of mutual destruction. 'The whole family calls him Bruce. It helps us to deal with it,' his owner explained, and again I remembered his dry humour of old, smoothing awkward moments in a consultation and implying 'You and I are both in on this joke' to cement the therapeutic relationship.

Having been introduced to Bruce, it was only polite to give him some attention. He rose like a rugby ball from the lower left part of his owner's belly, as hard as a rock and overlaid by stretched, shiny white skin bearing distended blood vessels like a tattoo of rats' tails. Bruce was exquisitely tender to the touch, and the pain drained the remaining colour from my patient's face. I cannot say that I was pleased to make Bruce's acquaintance. However, the moment of shared humour opened up a new spirit of understanding, and I was allowed to talk about pain relief.

Like partners in a courtly dance, we explored his experience of morphine together. He knew it only as a drug of abuse from his psychiatric practice. As a junior doctor he had been familiar with the 'Brompton cocktail', a brew that was concocted to manage intractable cancer discomfort before we understood pain well, and before we had worked out how to titrate painkillers so that they matched the individual patient's pain and left their mind clear. In those days rendering a patient unconscious was considered an act of kindness, he said, and the semi-conscious were unable to converse in any intelligent way while taking this industrial-strength drug mixture.

Of course, I accepted his premise that seeing him thus mentally incapacitated would be very distressing for his family, and would undermine his own sense of personal dignity. In return, he accepted that I had some experience of using these drugs very carefully, and had even undertaken several years' training to become a consultant in palliative medicine, a specialty only invented in the 1980s. Perhaps he might allow that medicine had progressed since the Brompton cocktail. And with this mutually gracious exchange, he agreed to a cautious experiment with a very small dose of morphine. Over the next three days he allowed us to increase the dose, and we watched his deckchair posture unfold, until I met him walking along the hospice corridor, glowing with the joy of freedom from pain.

He was delighted with the hospice. He admired everything, and I remembered that this had always been his way. He thanked the nurses and praised the cleaners and asked the chef to visit for personal congratulation. He was constantly attended by members of his loving family, a wife and three daughters and occasionally several small grandchildren whom he held in thrall with his story-telling. As his pain improved, giggles of delight and gasps of excitement rang from his room as he told them his tales. With his pain better controlled, he was able to return to light duties as a climbing frame, which is a very important grandpaternal role. 'Everyone just has to be careful not to nudge Bruce.'

I often popped in to see him at the end of my working day, and on one of those occasions he explained to me his deep lone-liness. Since he had realised that he was dying, he was no longer able to indulge his lifelong love of the music of Mahler. The pathos and beauty of the music now resonated too deeply with his sense of approaching farewell. He found the time between family visits hung heavy in the absence of his beloved music. His dignity in revealing his soul in this way was immense, and we sat in silence together, contemplating those ideas so huge that words will not suffice.

Along the corridor, a secret musician was also approaching the end of her life. She was a feisty widow who had brought up two sons alone; she had worked as a hospital cleaner, and at night-time she topped up her income with bar work. Her sons described her as strong, proud and funny. Her anecdotes from her barmaid days kept us all entertained, and were expressed in a breathless wheeze of colourful language and local dialect. She had a chest condition that had gradually contracted all her horizons – confined to walking short distances, then to home, then to a chair, and now to bed. Because of paroxysms of unpredictable breathlessness, at home she slept with a phone beside her bed, but when she dialled her sons they were unable to decipher her breathless panic. Her chest medicine team had referred her for hospice care in the hope that we could reduce the level of night-time panic associated with her breathlessness.

She managed her breathlessness by humming. She told us that she found it controlled the speed of her out-breath (*Try it!*) and gave her a sense of control. She favoured jazz tunes, of which she seemed to know an endless number. She told us that she had a collection of jazz tapes that she sang along to at home. Her breathlessness was worse at night because her very old cassette player had no headphones, so she didn't play it at night-time in case she disturbed her neighbours. She pressed her sons to bring some audiotapes and the precious tape recorder from home. It took them some time to excavate them from the chaos of a household where maintenance had become neglected as her chronic chest complaint had made her too breathless for housework.

The tapes were a mixture of Ella Fitzgerald and Billie Holliday, and some live recordings from a noisy bar of a singer with a breathtaking voice. This, she explained, had been her 'untapped' career: she had been a jazz singer on cruise ships when she met her husband, but had given up singing to keep his house and rear their children. The boys had never known her as a singer; she had stopped singing as a young widow when the light in her voice was extinguished by sorrow. Only recently had she returned to her music for solace as her breathing failed.

'Billie-Ella', as the nurses admiringly dubbed her, played these tapes constantly, sometimes listening to her heroines and sometimes replaying her own voice and reminiscing about those happy, heady days of her courtship and early marriage. She hummed along as best she could, breathing deeply between bars, assisted by piped oxygen. Her sons were stunned to realise that their mother had such a talent, and such encyclopaedic knowledge of jazz. The nurses were astonished by how much better she tolerated her breathlessness when the music was playing.

The hospice's acoustics carried the music to her neighbour's room at night-time, and on one of my end-of-day visits he commented that since he started the morphine, his sleeplessness had been comforted by a kind of 'dreamy singing'. He had never heard music like this before, and spent several nights wondering whether his medications were causing some kind of hallucination. He was delighted when the night nurses assured him that the music was real, and he asked them to sit him in the corridor so he could listen more intently.

And so the doctor and the barmaid were introduced. He knew very little about jazz, yet he quickly recognised that he was in the presence of greatness. Billie-Ella was delighted to play her tapes to someone who appreciated the velvet warmth of her youthful voice and the poignant jazz melodies of love and loss; her new companion found a new musical comfort that carried him through the absence of Mahler; and the two created a short, intense and mutually supportive friendship as they mentally jazz-danced through their final weeks of life. I was struck by the parallel lives they had lived in their love of music, albeit of very different genres, in their dedication to their families, in serving the NHS in two vital roles. It almost felt that their meeting at the edges of their lives was destined.

I don't go to many of my patients' funerals – it could become a regular occupation in my job. But I did feel a special tie with my erstwhile trainer, and I recognised many of our local medical confraternity at the crematorium when I arrived for his funeral service. We stood as the family arrived and the coffin was brought in to a passage from Mahler's 5th Symphony. There were many happy anecdotes about a man who had lived a full and largely happy life. And, as so often at funerals, we discovered that the wonderful man we had known was only the visible tip of the iceberg of his total being: he had taken homeless young people into his own home, rowed for his university, set up one of the first teenagers' psychiatry practices in the country, played viola in a semi-professional orchestra (*Ah! That adagietto in Mahler's 5th!*). As the coffin was removed and we stood to leave the celebration of his life, a solo jazz trumpet introduced the strains of Billie Holliday, his latest, and last, new passion. It sounded like Billie Holliday. Or perhaps it was our barmaid jazz singer.

Deep Dreams

I wrote this story shortly after the events took place, now many years ago. I was then a young doctor, married and a young mum myself, and I had a lot to learn about life. It seems to me still that this family taught me many things, in a series of chapters.

So here's a thing. I first looked after Pete when his rare cancer was newly diagnosed and operated on more than half a decade ago. He was a handsome young husband and father of two small boys who believed he was invincible. And since his outlook was very poor, and this is six years later, he almost was. His experience was one of the events that turned my career intentions towards cancer management and palliative care. I have thought of him, of his tiny, strong wife and of their beautiful, innocent boys, many times since I looked after him on a surgical ward a few months after I qualified as a doctor.

Let me give you the back story. Pete was a deep-sea diver who worked away from home for weeks at a time. When he was home he was a dedicated dad, a keen member of a five-a-side football team, and had a personal seat at his favourite pub, where he and his former school friends swapped stories about their lives: the coalmines, shipbuilding, oil and gas, the heavy industries that absorbed pimply youths in our area and turned them into old men. Pete was never a pimply youth. He was the local pin-up, and many hearts were broken when he married his childhood sweetheart Lucy. Pete was engaging and charismatic; he had the confidence of a man who knows himself to be attractive. The nurses would linger when offering him medications or meals. He met us all with a smile of his crinkly turquoise eyes.

But he was having trouble passing urine, and investigations showed that this was because he had a growth near his bladder. In the operating theatre all those years ago, when the surgeon got into Pete's pelvis, he found a huge tumour, and in cutting away as much of the mass as he could, he feared that he may have damaged some of the nerves that enable a man to control his bladder and to enjoy a sex life. This was going to be difficult news to break. It was broken the following day by the surgeon ushering all the female members of his ward round (which meant everyone except him) out of Pete's room, and then, as he left the room himself, with his hand on the door handle, turning back to Pete and Lucy and declaring, 'And by the way, you'll probably be impotent,' before closing the door behind him. The shock on their faces was the last thing I saw as the door closed, and in my head a different door opened, to the land of 'Medicine need not be like this.' The flame was lit for a career in communicating.

Pete's tumour turned out to be a very rare type, that can grow very big where it starts, and can also send tiny seeds out into other parts of the body, particularly the lungs. If caught early enough and completely removed, it can sometimes be cured. Pete's chest X-ray was clear, his whole-body CT scan was clear (that was an exciting new test at the time), and the surgeon hoped that the radical surgery, although possibly condemning Pete to a lifetime wearing a catheter and unable to have erections, might have been curative. Two weeks after the operation, with his catheter still in, Pete was allowed home for weekend leave. He was impishly delighted to report on his return to the hospital that 'that other thing' was fine: 'In full working order,' he beamed at me and a blushing nurse. She ran away. He winked. Lucy reached for his hand. I could feel my tears welling as I left the room.

Three months later Pete was back at work. He did not need a catheter, his sex life was 'top-notch', and he would be allowed to dive again six months after his surgery. He was tanned, beaming and confident, but Lucy, sitting beside him in the out-patient clinic holding his hand, looked strained and anxious, vigilant for any possibility of bad news. The chest X-ray was still clear. As she relaxed and smiled, I could see why he had fallen in love with her.

Wind forward six years. Prompted partly by that early experience, I am training in palliative medicine. My consultant trainer asks me if I can work late to visit a patient at home at the request of a local Macmillan nurse who is struggling to manage the pain of a young man with a rare type of cancer, pressing on his pelvic nerves. He tells me the name. My heart thuds and my stomach drops. I see Pete and Lucy's faces through that closing door so long ago, and my heart aches for them again. The home visit is arranged.

Lucy's eyes are full of tears as she opens the front door. 'I couldn't believe it was you when the nurse told me. Pete's so excited. The boys remember colouring in with you at the hospital.' She is even smaller than I remembered, and wound tight like coiled wire, mouth flat and drawn, clothes baggy on her tiny frame. She leads me upstairs, where a wasted, sallow man with Pete's brilliant eyes above hollow cheeks is sitting in striped pyjamas. A Belsen lookalike, I think, and then banish that thought as he smiles and the years drop away.

Pete resurrects that old joke. 'Still top-notch,' he tells me, 'but I don't have the energy and I lose my breath easily.' He has had lung secondary tumours for two years. Chemotherapy has thinned his hair but only partially shrunk his cancer. The last round of chemo had no effect, and there are no further options for shrinking his cancers. The Macmillan nurse has become involved because regrowth of the pelvic tumour (damn! a microscopic amount escaped the surgeon's knife and has regrown) is now compressing those delicate nerves in the pelvis, causing pain in Pete's bottom and legs. The tumour is getting bigger, and is pressing on some blood vessels. This has caused Pete's legs to retain water and become swollen, heavy. He struggles to manage the stairs, and has been living upstairs for the last two weeks.

We talk tactics, Pete and Lucy, the nurse and me. Pain caused by nerve damage is quite tricky to treat, and managing the swelling will involve bandaging his legs daily for a week or so until they go down enough for him to wear compression stockings. 'Very sexy,' he says, grinning. We three women are past the blushing stage of life. He agrees to a short hospice admission to sort out his leg swelling and try to get to grips with the pain. We may be able to improve his mobility, and if we can, he would like to take his boys fishing.

And so now here we are. Pete is once again a patient in my care, Lucy rushing between their home, where she sees the boys out to school and welcomes them home, and the hospice, where she spends the day sitting in Pete's room, searching his face for clues to his deepest thoughts while he limits any conversation to fishing, football and diving exploits from his exciting career. 'It's as though none of this is happening,' she tells me. 'As though he doesn't realise how sick he is. I don't know what to tell the boys. I don't know what to tell his mum. I don't even know what to think myself. I'm swinging between hoping for a miracle, and knowing that he's going to die. I'm completely lost.'

The leg swelling responds well to daily bandaging, and Pete's sense of humour ensures that the bandaging sessions are hilarious as he runs a commentary on the unwrapping and rewrapping, the gradual re-emergence of his kneecaps from the cylindrical, swollen limbs, the eventual reappearance of his toes from the bulging swelling in his feet, and the music-hall punnery of the swelling of his scrotum. The pain, however, is more of a challenge. The nerves in Pete's pelvis are under pressure from the tumour, and this sends waves of pain like electric shocks down the nerves into his legs and buttocks that leave him grey and exhausted every time he tries to stand up. Our drugs make very little difference; a combination of painkillers that might sedate a horse has simply enabled Pete to sit in bed with less discomfort, but with no prospect of walking or taking his sons out anywhere.

The boys visit in the evenings after school. Pete takes extra painkillers before they arrive, and insists on being helped into a chair so they don't see him in bed and become concerned. They bring their homework, they bring comic books, and they watch TV with their dad. Then Lucy takes them home and Pete goes back to bed, takes his evening pills and settles into sleep.

Except that he doesn't settle. In his sleep, Pete thrashes and shouts. He moves and grimaces. He awakens, sweating and breathless, shaking and afraid. On several occasions the on-call doctor has been sent for because the nursing staff were worried that Pete was having some kind of heart attack, or was struggling to breathe because of blood clots in his lungs, but his chest is physically unchanged when we examine him. It seems that he is having nightmares, yet afterwards he has no memory of them. He begins to dread night-time and to postpone going to sleep, with the result that he looks ever more exhausted by day, and his pain is getting worse.

One night, as Pete lies thrashing and calling out in his sleep, the night ward sister wakes him up mid-dream. He awakens shouting and waving his arms, then gradually calms as he recognises the half-lit room around him and the nurse sitting in the bedside chair. She asks if he can remember what he was dreaming about. Yes, he can. Yes, he can, and he now realises that this dream is the same, or very similar, every night. This dream terrifies him. It takes him back to his deep diving days. It brings him to the edge of his life.

Divers always work in pairs, Pete explains to the nurse. 'We must always be able to see each other. If something goes wrong, we're responsible for helping our "buddy" to the surface. We never abandon each other – it's a matter of principle, of honour, of sharing each other's danger below the water.' In the dreams, Pete and his long-term diving buddy are always on a deep dive, mending a pipeline in dark and dangerous waters. They are working some distance from each other when Pete realises that his oxygen tank is nearly empty. He has enough oxygen left to get to the surface, or to get to his buddy and alert him, but not to do both. He cannot surface and desert his buddy, even though it may cost him his life. But if he uses his oxygen to swim to his buddy, he will not be able to reach the surface. He cannot decide what to do. And while he struggles with the dilemma, his oxygen runs out. He is about to die. At that moment he always wakes in a breathless panic, yet unable to grasp the thread of the passing dream.

The nurse helps Pete to sit up. She turns the lights on, and makes a warm milky drink. And then she asks him what he thinks his dream is really about. He says, 'It's about diving. It's every diver's nightmare.'

She nods before saying, 'And could it be about anything else, Pete?'

Pete reflects. He nods and looks at the nurse. He tells her that the dream is about him, about Lucy, about dying. 'I can't leave her alone with the boys and all the things we should be dealing with together,' he says, 'but I can't help it. My time is running out. I'm going to die. She'll be alone with everything to deal with. I'm abandoning her. She is my dearest and best buddy, and I'm leaving her on her own.'

The nurse and Pete take time to digest this revelation. Pete is devastated by the reality he has been trying to ignore, the odds he has been trying to beat.

And then the nurse asks him what plan he might make to support Lucy. It is as though she has turned on a light beneath the waves and asked him to notice the diving bell that is available for both of them to be brought to the surface.

Pete leans forward and says, 'I have to help her now. We need to tell the kids. We need to do it together. I need to be at home. I need to support her. I need to sort out the mortgage and the insurance. We need to clear the garage. We need to be a team again. She doesn't have to do it all on her own . . . but she doesn't know that. Until I tell her.'

The night sister reported these events in her handover report next morning. But that didn't really prepare any of us for what happened next. Pete asked for a member of the ward team to help him explain to Lucy how close to death he was. He knew that his strength was ebbing week by week, and that his life expectancy was likely to be weeks, perhaps a few months at most. He and Lucy spent the morning talking, weeping, planning, and asking advice from our 'family worker' about how to explain to the boys that their dad was dying.

That evening, they asked their sons what worries they had about their dad.

The younger boy, now eight, said, 'I think about what will happen if you never come home.'

The older son, ten, said, 'You're not going to get better this time, are you Dad?'

When Pete and Lucy gave them the space, the boys seemed already to know that Pete would not live to the year's end. Both had been locked in a lonely place where pretending everything would be fine was the only acceptable behaviour.

They wept. Pete told them, 'It's OK to cry. We men, we can cry and be strong at the same time. It's not only women. Your mum is the strongest person I've ever met, and she cries like a girl. So we can cry like men. And then it's time to get stuff done.'

That night, and for the next several nights that Pete remained at the hospice, he slept without nightmares. He awoke looking refreshed. His pain reduced. He began to walk. His long-idle legs were weak, and he needed a walking frame, which he decorated in the colours of his football team. Lucy brought the car on Saturday, and they took the boys fishing. On Monday Pete went home. The bed had been moved downstairs and it almost filled the living room, but they all sat on it together to watch TV. Pete's five-a-side team came round to sort out the garage under his close supervision. This seemed to involve quite a lot of beer and singing, but was achieved in a week.

Despite the enlargement of his tumour, Pete's pain was well controlled. He remained mobile until two weeks before he died, then stayed in bed and declared that he was 'captain' of the house, managing everything from 'the bridge'.

Sometimes, it seems, a pain in the body is actually a pain in the soul, a pain in the deepest part of our being, often without a name or any recognition. By diving into his dream with him, that nurse enabled Pete to heal his deepest hurt, and that healing allowed him to die in peace.

De Profundis

Amongst the population is a cohort of people whose quality of life is affected by the complex difficulties of multiple illnesses, long-term frailty and very limited life choices. Some of them were born with complicated disabilities, many others have acquired a collection of conditions during their lifetime, and of course the very oldest are often those who have the greatest number of life-limiting conditions. Some have entirely physical limitations; some have conditions affecting their ability to think and respond; some have both.

The seriously sick, and the chronically frail, live altered lifestyles with plenty of time to contemplate the impact of the changes in their lives. Some who look exhausted retain an inner vigour and zest for life; some who seem relatively well are unbearably challenged by the loss of their previous fitness. Only by listening to these people can we understand their perspective on living with illness, disability or frailty. Each is like a book recording a rich life story, that cannot be judged simply by its cover.

My son is playing his favourite music, an eclectic mix of Beethoven and banging beats. Struggling with my paperwork, I am hot and bothered. *Can't he use earphones?* As I prepare to negotiate, I am transported to another room, a decade ago, and a different blaring radio. Time slips away; I am back in the hospital ward with Mrs Liang, her radio, and her noisy neighbours.

Mrs Liang was ninety-eight years old. She grew up in Malaysia, and came to the UK to study as a young woman, at a time when few British women and even fewer Malaysian women took degrees.

As a professor of economics she wrote a world-changing book about debt and the developing world. This was a woman with a mighty mind.

She retired at seventy, but continued to campaign about Third World debt, addressing international meetings until her early eighties, when her husband died. After that Mrs Liang – Professor Liang – was alone. Her health began to fail. She had osteoporosis, and the thinning of her bones led to a series of painful fractures in her spine that reduced her height, bent her forward and limited her mobility. Poor circulation caused by diabetes led to ulcers around her ankles that confined her to a bed or chair. In her nineties she developed cataracts that prevented her from reading, which had been her passion, and she opted to move into nursing home care because she was unable to bathe, feed herself or get in and out of bed without help. At ninety-five she developed a tremor in her hands, and Parkinson's disease was diagnosed. The tremor meant she could no longer use utensils to feed herself, or use her radio unaided. She had been slowly losing weight over a few years. Her mighty mind was carried in a body that was wearing out. She was known to our hospital's diabetes clinic, neurology team and musculoskeletal service, but none of these departments could meet all of her needs.

I first met her when she was admitted to hospital via the emergency department, where her nurse asked for palliative care advice. Monique, one of our nurse specialists, and I went to ED to assess her.

The ED nurse, Maria, explained that our advice was needed about an elderly lady with pain in her back who had started screaming, which was upsetting the other patients in her bay. 'She's obviously upset, but we can't communicate with her,' said Maria. 'There's a carer with her from her nursing home, but she says this happens from time to time and they never know what to do either.'

Maria recites Mrs Liang's enormous drugs list: treatments for high blood pressure, for underactive thyroid, for her thinning bones, for her Parkinson's disease. It is a struggle to eat, but every day she must swallow three or four small 'meals' of pills.

Maria nods as Monique comments on the pills problem. I am reminded of an elderly woman I looked after as a very newly qualified doctor, who had a similar list of multiple ailments and associated remedies. 'How do you remember to take them all?' I had asked her, having diligently written down the formidable list of water tablets, heart pills, steroids and vitamins in the morning, more heart tablets and a thyroid pill mid-day, steroid at a lower dose, plus more heart pills late afternoon, and an assortment of other medications at bedtime. More than thirty different tablets every day.

She had winked at me with a puckish grin, then asked me to pull her shopping bag out of her bedside cabinet. Sitting forward on the bed, she unzipped the bag and extracted a huge glass jar, sold by a famous brand of confectioners for their Christmas selection, that was one third full of a pick-and-mix variety of loose tablets. I recognised the purple thyroid pills and some capsules for blood pressure amongst myriad white, blue, yellow and pink pills: discs, lozenges, squares and tiny spheres, some plain and others with letters or numbers stamped onto them.

'Each time I get a new prescription,' she confided to me, 'I open the bottles and tip all the pills into here. Then, four times a day, I pick out a handful and take them. It seems to work!' And indeed, it had worked for many months, until her random selection had not supplied enough of the tiny white Digoxin tablets needed to keep her heart in a steady rhythm and she ended up in hospital. I remembered how I had wished I could photograph that jar. I knew it illustrated a really important lesson about the dangers of polypharmacy – not just that the more drugs we prescribe, the more scope there is for error or interactions between them, but also that prescribing has to be realistic about a patient's lifestyle and ability or willingness to take their medications.

Now, here in the emergency department twenty years later, is a woman struggling to swallow who, instead of using that limited ability for pleasure, is subject to a daily battle to take her medicines and is probably left exhausted by the effort. No wonder she is screaming. Monique and I leave Maria to deal with a telephone query, and set off to find our patient.

There is a big name-board in the staff area, but we don't need it. The sound of a wailing, distressed patient fills the corridor, and we follow the sound to a bay where three women attached to drips and heart monitor wires are gazing forlornly at the curtains drawn around the fourth bed, from where the unhappy sound of shrieks, wails and grunts is emanating. Inside the curtains, a uniformed carer from a local nursing home sits in a plastic chair, speaking gently and calmly to the occupant of the bed – the famous economist.

Our patient hardly looks human. She is propped upright against pillows, but the curvature of her spine bends her chest forward so that her face is looking towards the mattress. Her legs are bent up and fixed by muscle contractures. Her pewter hair, still thick, hangs lank and matted. Her hands tremble restlessly in her lap. She could not look more different from my lively and mischievous pill-pooler of twenty years ago. Monique and I exchange glances. This is going to be a very challenging referral.

Monique goes into action. She kneels down beside the bed, so that she can look upward into Mrs Liang's face. She smiles and reaches out to stroke one of her hands, speaking slowly and gently. 'Hello, Mrs Liang. I'm Monique. I'm a nurse here . . .' Mrs Liang pauses, surprised, mid-wail, and locks her eyes on Monique. 'Hello,' smiles Monique again, as eye contact is held. 'Good to meet you.' Mrs Liang gives a single, doll-like blink, and holds Monique's gaze with the expressionless face of Parkinson's disease. 'You don't sound comfortable,' Monique continues, and Mrs Liang clumsily pats her abdomen with one trembling hand.

'She's had a tummy ache and been constipated,' the carer

explains, 'and our GP sent her in to get sorted out. But she hates sitting up leaning on her back. And she's anxious about leaving her own room. That's why I've come with her. I've brought her favourite blanket too.' She introduces herself as Doreen, and her eyes spill tears as she says, with surprising frankness, 'Sometimes they live too long, don't they? This isn't the way to live. Poor thing, and she's such a nice lady.'

Monique greets Doreen as a colleague, and immediately recruits her help. Doreen explains her charge's preferred reclining position, and with expert sliding of sheets, moving of pillows and gentle reassurance, Monique leads us through turning Mrs Liang onto her side, her limbs and curved spine now supported by plumped and folded pillows. Mrs Liang gives another slow blink, and her eyes crinkle at the edges.

'Aw, that's how she smiles!' exclaims Doreen, grasping Mrs Liang's hand. Mrs Liang takes a deep breath. She assumes a thoughtful expression, then whispers, 'Thank you.' It seems a great effort for her.

'Thanks for letting us move you,' says Monique, who then introduces me, as always, as her 'pet doctor'. She warns Mrs Liang that I may want to ask her a few questions, and Mrs Liang promptly closes her eyes.

Monique and I swap places, so I can stand where Mrs Liang can see me if she chooses to look. She is skeletally thin. There is a small break in the skin over her right shin, typical of the ulcers caused by poor circulation. The skin over the bony prominences at her ankles, knees, wrists and elbows is tight and shiny, but intact, a tribute to excellent nursing care at her home. I know we will need to examine the skin over her spine and sacrum too, but just now we will focus on what is easy for her, and complete our assessment gradually.

I contemplate our patient's predicament. This is extreme old age: frailty of body, multiplicity of health problems, loneliness at outliving friends and family, each factor impacting on the others and undermining the person's ability to engage fully with the world. This once mighty woman seems to be reduced to a husk. It's a truth rarely acknowledged that as we live longer thanks to modern medicine, it is our years of old age that are extended, not our years of youth and vigour. What are we doing to ourselves?

But tomorrow we can contemplate quality of life; today we have a pain to manage.

'I heard that your tummy is sore,' I begin, and Mrs Liang opens her eyes warily. 'I'd like to make it better if I can. Please will you hold my hand while I feel your tummy, and just squeeze if you need me to stop? I don't want to hurt you . . .' She holds my right wrist as I palpate her abdomen, as gently as I can, with my fingers. She allows me to continue, aware of where I will touch her because her hand is moving with mine. She is so thin, I can feel her organs with ease, and the utterly constipated intestine that explains her tummy pain.

Maria reappears through the curtains to announce that Mrs Liang has been allocated a bed on a care of the elderly ward. This is excellent news; her multiple challenging conditions will be viewed together and a plan of action made. The bed will be available in an hour. Monique and I suggest a management plan for resting her bowel and softening her faeces to stop her terrible cramping pains; after a day or two of rested bowel and softening agents, the nurses on her new ward will be able to help her move her bowels far more comfortably. Her stiff, trembling muscles may yet respond to a review of her Parkinson's medications. Perhaps she will go home slightly better than she arrived here; it's a game of diminishing returns, and any small improvement may make a big difference.

I follow Mrs Liang's progress on the COTE ward via Monique, who visits her daily to assess the impact of the bowel management plan. She is being nursed on a special mattress to protect her skin; her constipation is resolving; her pain is under control. Her drugs have been considerably reduced, and some tablets have been replaced by skin patches so there are fewer to swallow. Her tremor is less, although her facial expression remains fairly blank. Plans are being made to get her back to her nursing home, but she continues to have a pain in her right foot that is causing concern, and Monique has asked for my opinion about it.

When I arrive it is just after lunchtime. The patients' meals are being cleared away, and Mrs Liang is sitting in a reclining chair, resting on her back (a prize of better pain control) and tilted backwards so she can face towards the window instead of the floor. There is a radio playing classical music on her table, and I ask her permission to turn it off briefly so we can talk.

'I wish someone would throw it out of the window!' she replies, unexpectedly loudly, reaching her trembling arm towards it. 'Noisy damn thing. They leave it on all day, and it drives me mad!' I have often noticed the tendency to have background music in hospital and care homes, and wondered who makes the choices.

'Do you prefer peace and quiet? Or are you a talk radio listener?' I ask her, and she tells me she loves BBC Radio 4, which 'treats me like I have a brain'. I assure her that after our talk I will retune the radio for her. With a slow blink, she tells me that Monique retunes it each time she visits, but the other women in the six-bedded bay complain that the talking interferes with their enjoyment of their music. 'Many of these women are hard of hearing,' she says, 'or unable to manage those earphones, so all are compelled to listen, at high volume, to the choice of one individual. Dante would have mentioned this punishment had radio been invented when he was describing the Inferno.'

Looking around the room, I take in five other elderly women. All are clad in clean but garish hospital gowns. Their fitter fellow patients are helped to dress in daywear, but this room houses the most frail members of the ward. Some are sleeping gently. One holds up a hand towards me as though she hopes I might rescue her. Another is carefully holding a plastic, spout-mouthed cup with focused attention. A contemporary *Inferno* might also have described this scenario: the vicissitudes of extreme age, of a clear mind being tied to an existence that crumbles in staccato steps yet continues to be experienced; or life no longer experienced in abundance by those with inexorable cognitive decline but cruelly robust physiques. This room could be a very clean and tidy Circle of Hell, and it would be easy to suppose that these women would greet death as a welcome guest.

And yet, what can seem intolerable to the observer is often counted as life worth living by the elderly. Mrs Liang did not suddenly wake up old one day; she arrived here via a long and gradual journey of stepwise dwindling, occasional partial recoveries, intermittent thrusts of illness and parries of treatment. She and I observe her situation from entirely different vantage points, and it is her interpretation that counts. As I spend more time with elderly people, I am learning not to make assumptions.

I sit down beside her to discuss how things are progressing. She is delighted that her tummy pain is settled and her constipation resolved. The stronger painkillers allow her to lie on her back, in a position that makes it easier to see the world despite the continued crumbling of her spine. She has had her hair washed, combed and cut by the hospital hairdresser, and the rehabilitation team has provided large-grip utensils that enable her to feed herself, although her Parkinson's disease makes her so slow that she needs help, and she has agreed to have a feeding tube placed to help her to maintain nutrition with far less effort. Better nutrition will protect her skin, and her drugs can be squirted down the tube instead of all that effortful swallowing. She will be able to eat and drink small amounts as she wishes, simply for the pleasure of it. This sounds appealing to her.

'I have lived too long,' she tells me, without emotion, in an echo of the words spoken by her carer on the day of her admission. 'If I could, I would give some of my years to younger people, people with families, people who need to live longer but can't.' If only length of life were as simple as a transferable asset. This is an economics assessment of the predicament in which she finds herself.

'Do you wish to be dead?' I ask her, and she pauses to think before telling me that she does not wish deliberately to end her life, but regrets that she has lived past being useful and mobile. I nod, and reflect that she is naming a key difficulty of older age.

I am about to turn to the subject of the pain in her foot when I suddenly become aware of a sense of heat. I am burning, radiating warmth and feeling the disconcerting, panic-like disquiet that accompanies menopausal flushing. I know that my face will be blushing, and I can feel my body perspiring.

Mrs Liang indicates what looks like a spectacles case on her tabletop, and asks me to open it. Inside is a battery-operated hand-held fan. She squeezes the handle to start it, and points it at my face, saying, 'Don't worry, dear. They pass very quickly, but aren't they a nuisance?' She waits for the flush to pass, watching my face intently as she fans me. I am overcome by this act of kindness, this simple acknowledgement of our biological sisterhood.

'I used to find them such a problem,' she tells me, 'because all the other people in my university department were men. Nobody understood. There, do you feel better?' I nod gratefully, and she squeezes the handle to turn off the fan.

'One gets used to them eventually,' she says. 'And yes, it's lovely when they stop! I don't miss them.' She tells me that her flushes stopped in her mid-eighties – I hope my face does not betray the horror of my inner calculations. This is when I sense that something interesting has happened: our relationship has shifted. Now, an older woman is mentoring a younger one. Mrs Liang's aged body still contains an agile mind that wants to keep abreast of current affairs; that has developed an economics-based philosophy of time passing; that has wisdom to impart and kindness to dispense, and yet very little opportunity to do so. In her simple act of compassion, she has been momentarily whole again.

The foot pain is easy. She tells me it feels like cramp, and when I examine it I see the sharp edge of a strap-like muscle pulling across the arch of her foot. She is quite correct; this cramp is a recognised feature of Parkinson's disease, and can probably be managed using a Botox injection to paralyse the muscle for a few weeks or months, repeated as needed. No need for extra painkillers, no sudden cramps to disturb her peace of mind or her sleep.

She tells me what wavelength Radio 4 is on and I retune her radio, propping it beside her ear on her pillow so she can hear but the other patients will not. We chuckle like co-conspirators. I stand to leave. The women around us look somehow different; I feel an awareness of our similarities, rather than of the differences imposed by age and ill-health. Our elderly are so easily dispossessed, stripped of their personhood by eyes like mine too young to value their accumulated wisdom, experience and patience. I have learned an important lesson from this very frail and aged woman.

'Goodbye, my dear,' she murmurs in valediction.

'Goodbye, and thanks, Prof,' I reply.

She gives that doll-like blink, and her eyes crinkle at the corners. We have done each other good.

The quality of an individual's life can really only be measured by that person. It is very easy to assume that living with illness becomes a burden, yet the elderly often accept their physical limitations as a price worth paying for living longer. Loneliness, many tell us, is a far harder burden than ill-health, and this is a sadness hidden in plain sight, a modern epidemic.

The price of living longer is that we experience older age, with or without cognitive decline. In 2015, for the first time ever, dementia became the commonest cause of death in England, although this reflects better data-collection as well as the increasing incidence of dementia. The rise of dementia is a moral and social challenge for the developed world, where families are scattered and the elderly are less likely to live with relatives.

How we deal with the most vulnerable members of our society is a true test of our values. Having accepted their contribution to the public good during their working lives, how should we support these weary elders? How do we enable them to experience satisfaction and self-worth, not in return for making a contribution, but simply for being their unique selves?

Perfect Day

Words are immensely powerful. When we talk, we assume that our listener interprets our words in the same way that we intended them, yet this may not always be the case. Misunderstanding based on different interpretations is even more likely when cultural differences are at play. It may not be our words, but their unintended meaning, that is heard. This may cause hurt and confusion, but it may also open up new possibilities that we had not anticipated – especially if we had felt lost for words, and thereby communicated our own vulnerability and common humanity to our listener.

It's a windy day, and wrinkled, nut-brown leaves are scuttling across the car park like a mischief of excited mice as I rush into the hospice at lunchtime. I have too many bags, as usual – my briefcase, a backpack and a large shopping bag containing last night's paperwork. My children think that my secretary marks my homework.

Crashing clumsily into the clerical office I can see pewter-grey clouds scudding along the sky over the river valley that drops below us – there will be autumn rain before the end of the day. Did the children take coats to school? I can't remember. I present a tape of dictated letters and a list of appointments and phone calls for my much-appreciated secretary to work through, explain the contents of the shopping bag, and run downstairs, where the team is assembling to discuss our patients before we begin our ward round.

So here we are: our ward sister, a social worker, a chaplain, a physiotherapist, a doctor spending six months with us as part of his GP training, a doctor who is training in palliative medicine and is nearly ready to apply for her first consultant job, and me. Our occupational therapist will join us when she can. She is baking cakes with a patient who cannot remember what she did yesterday, but who remembers baking with her mother many years ago. This kind of memory work often unlocks important new information in understanding our patients better. And it provides cake.

The meeting begins. One of my ward-round habits is that we have a cup of tea or coffee together while we talk through the important issues for our patients. Then, once we have discussed the main areas to be tackled during the ward round, we process around the hospice, visiting each patient in turn. For some, the focus may be a physical symptom or progress towards plans for home; for others it may be the effects of a recent change of medication, or the impact of work done in physiotherapy or occupational therapy sessions; for others again we may be discussing emotional distress or existential issues. Occasionally there is a new patient for me to meet, in which case the full story-so-far will be presented by one of the junior doctors, and we will consider the whole list of issues to be addressed for the patient and their family.

Today's meeting will discuss five current patients whom I know well, two more whom I have known from my work in the hospital palliative care liaison team and who have transferred to the hospice for attention to particular symptoms, and one new patient.

The new patient, Mrs Namrita Baht, is presented by our GP trainee. Namrita is thirty-seven years old. She is married with eight children, aged between sixteen and two. They are a devout Muslim family, and she observes prayer times at the hospice. She has lung cancer that has now spread to her liver, and this is causing her to feel very nauseated. She has been referred to the hospice by her GP, who found her vomiting into a bowl at home, surrounded by concerned relatives and her eight children, and thought we might be able to help to manage her symptoms and give her a chance to rest.

Namrita had agreed to come to the hospice. Her mother-in-law brings the children to visit by taxi every day. Her husband attends every evening after work. Her oldest daughter, Rubani, is sleeping at the hospice and acts as an interpreter for her mother, who speaks no English. What about the interpretation service, I ask. It seems callous to ask a sixteen-year-old to interpret conversations about her mother's serious illness. Namrita doesn't want an interpreter apart from family, the team assure me. Her nausea remains a terrible problem, but she declines to take any of the medicines that we would usually employ.

'Do we know why she won't take the medications?' I ask.

'We can't work it out,' says Sister. 'At first we thought she was afraid of the needle, but she won't try tablets for constipation or linctus for her cough either.'

'Does she think she should be using traditional medicines?' asks the chaplain.

'No, it's not that,' says Sister. 'It's as though she and her husband believe that she should be suffering. It's so sad to watch. She can't move in the bed without retching. Her youngest is only two, and he wants to sit on her knee, but Namrita has to keep the bowl on her knee. He sits on the knee of his grandma or one of his sisters, and just cries.'

'Sometimes devout Muslims will accept suffering as the will of Allah,' says the chaplain. 'It may be hard for us to watch, but this may be something that makes sense to her. That's worth asking about on the round.'

The meeting takes on a distinctly glum mood. We deal with suffering every day, all day, but our coping mechanism is to help. If our help is declined, we feel disempowered and our helplessness opens the gates to sadness.

We finish our no-longer-hot drinks and set off around the ward. Sister has asked Mr Baht to attend, and he will be here in an hour, so we review everyone else first.

By the time we reach Namrita's room, the chaplain has left us to visit a family who requested her help, and the OT has sent apologies because the bakery therapy has unlocked vast reminiscences for the forgetful patient, who is delighted that the rock buns taste exactly as she remembers them from childhood. There are only six of us in the procession, but it still feels numerous and awkward as we ask permission, and then file into the room.

Namrita is tall but wasted. She sits on her bed hunched and still, trying to overcome the waves of nausea storming her being. Her hijab remains in place even when she is retching and heaving into a bowl held by the nurses or by her calm daughter Rubani, who rubs her back, murmuring comfort in Punjabi and explaining Namrita's distress to us in English. Mr Baht sits on a low stool at the foot of the bed, running his fingers through his hair and frowning. The other children and their grandmother have gone to wait in the day room, respectful of the privacy they believe to be required when The Consultant attends.

I introduce the team, shake hands with Namrita and her husband, and move around the bed to sit in the upright armchair by the window. The rest of the team find places to sit. It's another of my ward-round habits that we all sit – it shows respect when we do not stand above the patient's eye level, and gives the tone of a visit rather than just 'popping in'. The single rooms are designed with a sofa-bed built into the wall, so four people can perch there. The others find chairs or sit on the floor. I'm usually a floor-sitter myself, but for this family I have the sense that etiquette is important, so I sit up straight and try to look like The Consultant.

We discuss Namrita's health journey so far. Her husband, Preetam, speaks fluent English with a song-like Punjabi accent. He explains that he cannot usually visit during the day because he must run his business. Rubani fills in some details: her father owns a flourishing carpet shop, and is a respected member of the local Pakistani community, the mosque and the mercantile confraternity. He supports his family in the UK and in Pakistan. She is clearly very proud of him. Work is an important duty for him, even though his wife is so sick. 'It breaks Daddy's heart to see her so sick,' Rubani tells us, 'and he cries sometimes.'

Mr Baht tells us that Namrita has been the treasured jewel of his life. He brought her to England for them to make their fortune selling rugs and carpets. Although a fortune has not quite been made, a happy and comfortable life has been lived amongst the Punjabi community, and Namrita has never felt a need to learn English. The family has grown, and most years they pay for relatives to visit them from Pakistan. They all enjoy extended visits from Namrita's sister and family, and from Preetam's parents. This was happily-ever-after.

Then, about a year ago, Namrita began feeling tired while she was breastfeeding her youngest child. She initially put it down to pregnancy, childbirth and her busy house, but as the baby was weaned her energy levels remained low, and she began to cough. Preetam's mother advised traditional medicines, but Preetam was a fan of the National Health Service, and insisted that Namrita should visit a GP.

Over a two-week period, Namrita was investigated and found to have an extensive lung cancer. Preetam attended all her clinic appointments, and translated what the doctors told her. They wept together with the kind chest physician when the diagnosis was made.

'That man seemed very kind,' Preetam says, 'but we were to find that he could not be trusted.'

I know the doctor he is describing, and I would trust him with my life. I wonder what happened. I wait for the story to unfold.

At all the hospital visits, Preetam translated Namrita's questions, and conveyed the doctors' answers to her. The cancer was too large for surgery, and she was offered a combination of chemotherapy and radiotherapy to shrink it, although the specialists in the cancer centre explained that this would not be a cure. Her best hope was that she might see her toddler start school.

Namrita entered a strange new world. She was admitted to the cancer centre, where she had radiotherapy several times each day, along with pulses of chemotherapy by drip. It was exhausting. She prayed constantly to become well enough to care for her family again, and gradually she began to cough less. She went home, where Preetam's mother had taken up residence to look after the children, and with love and home cooking she began to gain weight. Her hair regrew.

'She attended the school sports day and she looked so much better,' Preetam told us, 'until the sickness came. Feeling sick, like on a boat, all the time. Not eating. Vomiting. This was not good, and I realised that she needed help. We went back to the chest doctor, and he found that the cancer was now in her liver. Very bad. Very serious.'

He paused. We waited. He swallowed. He licked his dry lips and ran his fingers through his hair again, watching his exhausted wife retching while Sister held the bowl for her and wiped her face with a damp cloth. He was spent. My turn to talk.

'Mr Baht, we are so very glad to take care of Namrita,' I begin cautiously. He nods. 'I know she doesn't understand what I am saying, so please may I ask you to explain to her first that you have been telling me about how she got so sick?' He nods again, and speaks to his wife in Punjabi, while their daughter watches her mother's face with deep concern.

'And now, Mr Baht, I hope that you can help me to ask Namrita some questions, so that we can do our best to help her. Please will you explain that I would like to ask her some questions?'

Again, he speaks in gentle tones to his wife.

'What we would like to understand,' I say, 'is why Namrita, who feels so very sick, doesn't want to take the medications that we feel sure would help her.'

His body snaps upright in his seat, and he fixes me with a bright and focused stare. 'I can answer that for both of us,' he announces. 'We have realised that we cannot take any advice from

British doctors. No – none at all. For British doctors think that they are God. They think they know the mind of God. That is what we found with that doctor we trusted at the hospital. If doctors think that they are the equal of God, then they are misguided and we must not trust them.'

I am dumbfounded. I had not expected this. I think of my gentle, kind colleague at the hospital, who has managed this family with such diligence and attention. He would be astonished to hear this accusation. He is possibly the humblest man I know.

The heads of my colleagues, all previously turned towards Mr Baht, now swing towards me. Our experienced trainee has eyes like saucers; the social worker looks as if she is watching a suspense movie. They are waiting to hear my response.

'Thank you for telling me that,' I say in as measured a tone as I can. 'Please will you explain to Namrita what you just told me, so she knows what we are talking about?' He turns to her, and the gentle tones become more abrupt as they exchange a few phrases. He turns back to me.

'Thank you. It's good to know that Namrita knows what we are saying,' I say. 'And now, if you would be so kind, please will you help me to talk directly to Namrita?'

Turning towards her, I say, 'Namrita, I understand that you lost confidence in Dr O'Hare because he seemed to think he knew the mind of God. Have I understood you correctly?' Mr Baht repeats my question in Punjabi – I hope. I have no way of knowing, although Rubani seems content with the exchanges. Namrita says a few words, and Rubani waits for her father to translate, 'Indeed. We were very shocked.'

'Namrita, can you explain to me what happened that day?' I ask.

Her husband exchanges some phrases with her, and then Rubani says, 'Mummy says she is very tired. She suggests that Daddy will explain, and I will tell Mummy what he is saying.'

'Thank you, Namrita,' I say, keeping my gaze on her. 'You rest there, and we will let him explain.' Rubani whispers to her mother, while I turn back to Mr Baht, and the whole team turn their heads in unison towards him.

'We went to his clinic,' says Mr Baht, 'and we knew she was worse. We had discussed at home that she would want to die in Pakistan, the land of her birth, and to have the proper funeral observances there. So I said to the doctor at the clinic that I wanted to take her home to Pakistan.' He draws breath, giving Rubani time to whisper to her mother.

'But what do you think he said? He said her lungs could not cope in an aeroplane. So I told him we can travel by boat and by train. And *then* what do you think he said?' He pauses and looks at me expectantly. All heads in the room turn towards me.

'What did he say?' I ask quietly, and the heads swing back to face him.

'He said . . . He said . . . He told us that she will die before she gets there. That she will die in three months. That she cannot live longer than three months. But only God can give life or take it away. Only God! So if he thinks – if British doctors think – that they can know the mind of God, then we cannot accept their help. It is sacrilege. It cannot be so!'

The faces swing back to me. There is silence. Rubani is also silent, her eyes startled and tears on her cheeks. This is news to her. In his heated distress, her father has told her more than she previously knew. As Mr Baht holds my gaze with defiant anger, I can see from the corner of my eye that Sister is reaching out to take Rubani's hand. All faces gaze at me. And I understand how a cultural mismatch has undermined the trust between the Bahts and British medicine. Yet how on earth can I address it? *I have no words to put this right.*

'Oh, my goodness. I understand now why you don't feel you can take our advice. I can see how hurtful those words would be, even though I think he only intended to help you.' Pause. Gazes still on me. Eyes on stalks.

I imagine the pain of these good people, trying to live faithfully. What a terrible dilemma. What courage and self-denial. I can feel my throat tightening and tears welling. I struggle to keep my voice steady and calm.

'Mr Baht, Namrita, Rubani. I don't know what to say to you. I am so sorry that you should be so very hurt by a doctor who is my colleague and friend.' I pause, and Rubani whispers to her mother.

'All I know is that, while you are here, we will treat every day as a gift from God. Namrita is welcome to stay here, whether you can accept our medicines or not. Thank you for helping us to understand. Please tell Namrita how much I admire her courage to accept these awful symptoms.' Rubani whispers her translation, and Namrita stares at me across her vomit bowl and tries to smile, nodding.

'Is there anything else you would like to discuss while we are here?' I ask.

There is not. I stand. The team members and Mr Baht rise to their feet. The team leaves, and I shake hands again with the family before leaving. I am utterly exhausted by the exchange, and hopeless about being able to reduce Namrita's symptoms. We trudge back to the ward office in silence.

We take a ten-minute debrief before we all head on to our next tasks. The OT arrives (with rock buns) and we ponder how best to help the Baht family. Their faith is of central importance in their lives, and any attempt by us to challenge their interpretation of this situation may fracture our relationship with them, as it already has with the unwitting chest physician. We decide to ask our chaplain to call their mosque tomorrow and ask for advice, without naming names. The unused drugs remain prescribed and available at any time should Namrita change her mind.

'That was beautiful, what you said about every day being a gift from God,' reflects our social worker.

'I couldn't speak,' says our nearly-consultant doctor. 'I just felt overwhelmed by her predicament. I was agog to know what you would say.'

I tell them that I had no idea what to say either, so I just told them how we work here: every day is a new one, like a gift, and we try to make every day worthwhile. It's just what we do. I still feel overwhelmed, but it's time to do the school run and then go home to prepare supper, so I gather my wits and my bags and head out as the rain starts, blowing sideways in a miserable mist that suits my mood.

My daughter is a year older than Namrita's youngest son. Children always become skittish on windy days, and nursery is noisy and tumultuous when I arrive to claim my tiny artist clutching her painting of a dinosaur talking to a frog. We scurry like the leaf-mice back to the car, and zoom to my son's school, where football practice is drawing to a muddy close. He is flushed and excited, and has to sit on plastic bags in the car because he is so wet. This amuses both children immensely, and there is much merriment on the journey home towards a warm bath and then our meal with their daddy. They love our attic bathroom, feeling warm and bubbly while the rain pounds the windows and the wind howls around the chimney above us. They chatter about dinosaurs and whether or not all frogs speak the same language, and I watch and listen and laugh and chat and wonder how Namrita will ever again share this intimacy with her beloved children in the short time she has remaining.

The next afternoon the wind has stopped when I arrive at the hospice, and the wet pavement is littered with leaves shining yellow, red and tawny gold. As I enter the building I find a note in my tray from Sister: 'Please come downstairs to see me about Namrita.' My heart sinks.

But Sister looks upbeat. 'Come and see this,' she says, leading me along the ward corridor, past the delicious smells of the dinner trolley that remind me again of all the pleasures Namrita has lost to nausea. Sister pauses outside Namrita's open door. Inside I see

Grandma and Rubani sitting by the window, facing the door and chatting to each other. Moving position, I can see Namrita sitting in bed with her toddler on her knee. She is smiling and utterly absorbed in her conversation with him. She begins to sing and to bounce him on her knee. There is no vomit bowl in sight. How is this possible?

Rubani smiles at me, and speaks to her mother. Namrita looks up at me and smiles a glorious, joyous smile. I am speechless. She lifts her sleeve and shows me the place where a tiny needle is taped to her skin, and then I see the fine plastic tube and realise that she has a syringe-driver pump in place. She is taking the drugs for nausea.

'How . . .?' I cannot even frame the question.

'Yesterday evening,' says Sister, 'Mr Baht came back after he had taken the children home, and they talked, and then he came to the office to say that she would try the drugs we recommend, because we are respectful of God's gift of life. She had a priming dose, then we started the syringe-driver. She slept all night, kept her fruit juice down this morning, and ate a chapatti for lunch.'

Managing Namrita's nausea, while maintaining her sense of spiritual integrity, gave her back her life. She was able to return home and live amongst her beloved family. She died in her own bed ten weeks after the chest physician predicted that she would not live for three months. That was seventy days of being a wife, a mother, a householder, a lover of God as she understood him. Although she never returned to her homeland, she was surrounded by her devoted community, and in the traditional manner, she was buried before sunset the following day.

'Only the Good Die Young'

As we finish our tour of the facts of dying together, let's pause to look at a paradox that occurs daily in palliative care. Often, when we turn up on a ward, or take a referral for community palliative care team support, the staff ask, 'Why do you always come to see our most lovable patients? How do you get all the nicest people in your care?' And it feels like a truth: when we look around the hospice in-patient ward, and the day care attendees, or our case list for the hospital or community palliative care teams, we realise that these are all remarkable people. Are we just looking at the world through rose-tinted glasses? Or is there genuinely something special about people who realise that the end of their life is approaching?

I have spent a lifetime pondering this idea. And gradually, I have begun to see a pattern. It is, in fact, a truth that almost all of the people we have the privilege of meeting towards the end of their lives are extraordinary. They tolerate their symptoms with courage. They adjust their hope from avoiding death to embracing each day as death approaches. They can let go of the tyranny of planning and worrying about the future, and simply bask in the present. This was so eloquently expressed by the dying playwright Dennis Potter in his final broadcast interview, when he described his new-found discovery of the ordinary, appreciating the blossom on the plum tree outside his window as 'the whitest, frothiest, blossomest blossom that there ever could be, and I can see it'.

These people change the centre of their world from self to others. They focus on loving their loved ones, but that kindness also beams onto everyone else around them – their fellow patients in hospital or hospice, and all of us who care for them. They are the patients who notice that a nurse looks tired or remember that the cleaner's daughter is sitting exams. They express appreciation, concern and gratitude. And we bathe in the light of their beneficence.

What is going on here? What is the transformational catalyst that reshapes a grumpy retired coalminer or a previously pedantic professor into a somehow nobler version of themselves? The change does not extinguish their lifelong foibles, but in some way it smooths the roughest edges, so that our inept offerings of care and company are less likely to snag on a sharp temper or ignite an irascible ember. They have become, in some ineffable way, a bigger and more generous version of themselves, and the process is often invisible to them. They simply find that people around them are kinder, gentler, and with more forgivable faults than before. They don't see that this is a virtue of their own disposition; they credit the world around them for being a better place than they had previously believed.

In the world's wisdom traditions, from modern happiness experimental psychology, through the great faiths, and in the atheistic wisdom of Confucius and the stoic philosophers, much has been said about the growth of the inner person over a lifetime as we move towards wisdom. A human life of two parts is recognised in these traditions. The first part of life is establishing our identity and becoming a 'safe pair of hands' for adulthood. This first phase of life is, necessarily, egocentric. It is all about me. What am I about? What do I stand for? What are my gifts and talents, my strengths and capabilities? Does the world recognise my abilities? Perhaps there is some self-scrutiny to discern my faults and weaknesses, but that is only to ensure that I can hide them from the view and judgement of others. In this way, over the first part of a human lifetime, each of us identifies who we believe ourselves to be.

The second part of life is about transcendence to wisdom, and for many people this only develops over a long lifetime. For others, though, there can be an early transition, and this is very often through a personal experience of deep loss and enormous pain – exactly like the experience of knowing they have an incurable illness that our patients encounter; the knowledge that death is approaching, and that it will mean the end of everything they hold familiar and dear. Each of the wisdom traditions describes this transformation process in its own way, yet the key 'Golden Rule' of all of them is the development of a sense of compassion for others. The focus moves from 'me' to 'everyone and everything'. This includes a kindness to oneself, and the ability to recognise and forgive one's own faults in the same loving way that those transformed, second-part-of-life people forgive the faults of others.

The stories of the people facing death that I have shared in this book are mainly about people who have reached that new phase in their lives. They have become compassionate and wise, they overlook or even embrace the foibles of others, and they relish their sense of 'being' in every moment.

This transformation of world view is a spiritual transformation, whether theistic or not. It enables the person to review their life and to recognise and regret any hurt they may have caused other people, and often to desire to make amends. It is this recognition that underlies the first of the recurring last messages of dying people: 'I am sorry. Please forgive me.' It also supports their desire to avoid causing any further hurt, and this translates into a deeper patience with others' shortcomings.

Compassion also enables people to review personal hurts in a less judgemental way, and so the second of the last messages is often 'Don't worry about it. I forgive you. It is no longer a hurt between us.' Sometimes dying people seek out those from whom they have become estranged to offer a bridge of friendship. Time, distance or death may prevent this, yet the decision to forgive can still release the person from the hurt. This is powerful stuff.

The compassionate appreciation of others as people who are

only as flawed as the observer, and equally worthy, enables people to be deeply appreciative of those around them. People approaching the end of life are grateful for the tiniest kindness. They appreciate the good intentions behind often gauche expressions of support. They are grateful for the experience of each moment, like the 'blossomest blossom' of Dennis Potter. The need to express gratitude to others is another of the last messages. 'Thank you' is now a heartfelt statement of appreciation, not a mere courtesy.

The last and most frequent of the last messages is 'I love you.' This is now a statement of total appreciation for the beloved. True compassion recognises yet overlooks the imperfections in the beloved and in the relationship, and simply appreciates the intention to love and to be loving. The love is deepest for those who are dearest, but it bubbles over into even everyday encounters with strangers and staff. In palliative care we look after people who have reached a phase in their lives when they unconsciously radiate love.

So, of course these are the favourite patients on any ward. Of course it always seems that the best people are dying. These are just ordinary people, like the rest of us, but they are at an extraordinary place in their life journey, and all of us benefit from their compassion. They are not, in the main, 'saints'. They still have grumpy moments and periods of intense sadness, fear or anger about their fate. But they are examples of what we can all become: beacons of compassion, living in the moment, looking backwards with gratitude and forgiveness, and focused on the simple things that really matter.

It's like watching a rose unfurl to perfection. At the moment of its greatest glory it is on the brink of the curling of its petals, the explosion of its colours, and the casting of its magnificence into the wind.

Pause for Thought: Transcendence

We have worked through a lot of ideas to get to this point. But here are the really Big Ideas. The evidence is that we all reach the end of our lives with a mixture of satisfaction and regret over our experiences – and the time to adjust that balance is now. Every moment of our lives is 'now' as we live it. So what can we do that adjusts the balance towards satisfaction and away from regret, even while we are not anticipating the approach of death?

What are the values that guide your decisions in life? How well have you met your own expectations? Do you judge yourself with as much kindness as you judge other people? Is there any change you would like to make so that your way of life fits better with your values and beliefs? What first step could you take?

Thinking about the last messages, who would you like to thank? And what for? Is there a way to let them know of your gratitude? Can you write a letter? Send an email? Shout to the wind? Tell the story of your gratitude to someone who will join you in a moment of appreciation?

What about forgiveness? Whose forgiveness would you like to seek? And what for? Do you need to apologise to someone, or is it time to forgive yourself? How can you express your sense of regret? Perhaps it's time to make contact with someone, and to offer the first step towards reconciliation. Perhaps for some reason reconciliation is no longer possible. If so, can you think of a way to atone for your offence? If this is causing you great concern, consider talking to a counsellor or a chaplain – no religious belief is required to consult a chaplain, and they have great wisdom in matters of regret and forgiveness.

Perhaps you are the offended party. Is there anyone you would like to forgive? Does anyone need your reassurance that a past quarrel or misunderstanding is no longer a grievance between you? How might you let them know? Do you have a mutual friend who might take a message? Can you telephone or write? Can you get together or use video-links to share a chat? Or is it enough to decide to forgive, to let the hurt go and move on?

And then there is all that love to be communicated. Sure, you can leave letters and cards and material goods in your will. But it's so much more meaningful to say it in person, or to write now, and give them a chance to know that you love them while you are still here. For children and grandchildren, share your happiest memories by annotating photos and letting them see the collection of childish drawings and letters you have kept over the years. Write letters for their future big occasions: finishing school, starting work, graduation, getting married, special birthdays – and do that as well as, not instead of, telling them how much you love and treasure them right now.

If you are struggling to start, have a look at the letter template in the Resources section at the end of this book (pages 336-7). You could photocopy it and fill it in, or you could just use the words and add your own.

It's your life that you are working on finishing well. It's a mighty piece of work. Give it the attention and the time you deserve.

Last Words

After sitting at so many deathbeds, and accompanying the final parts of so many people's journeys, a peculiar familiarity with dying becomes a daily companion. Strangely, this is not a burden or a sadness, but a lightening of perspective and a joyful spark of hope, a consciousness that everything passes, whether good or bad, and the only time that we can really experience is this present, evanescent moment. This makes hard times slightly easier to bear, and good times immediately precious. Both happiness and disappointment will pass in time. Awareness of the temporary essence of all lived experience is humbling. That is why Roman generals who were granted a Triumph (a congratulatory public parade to mark their accomplishments) were accompanied in their chariot throughout the pomp and cheering by a slave whose role was to remind them of their mortality, and that this moment too will pass.

The folk stories of every society include quests for immortality that almost always come to a bad end. Or they tell of immortals whose deathless nature condemns them to loneliness. Or, most significantly of all, they speak of immortals who sacrifice their immortality to live a mortal life, for the love of a human being. The distillation of a civilisation's wisdom into its folk tales shows us that immortality is recognised as a poisoned chalice. Death itself is perceived by ancient wisdom as a necessary and even welcome component of the human condition: a finality that ends uncertainty or despair; a mandated temporal boundary that makes time and relationships priceless; a promise of the laying down of the burdens of living, and the end of the repeated daily struggle.

In sharing the stories of so many ordinary people as they reached their final days, I hope that I have shown that, in the end, none of us is ordinary, that each unique individual is extraordinary in their own way. As we approach the ends of our lives, we experience a shift in perspective that allows us to focus on the most important things in our own domain. This shift is both poignant and freeing, as these stories illustrate. Living is precious, and is perhaps best appreciated when we live with the end in mind.

It's time to talk about dying.

I have. Thank you for listening. Now it's your turn to talk.

Glossary

Every profession has its own language of technical words and abbreviations that make sense to co-workers but that may mystify the non-initiate. Wherever possible, I have tried to avoid medical jargon to allow the reader to understand what is unfolding even where the medical concepts are not simple.

However, there are non-technical words that will be familiar to users of British health services, but that may not be clear to non-British readers. Here are some terms I have used throughout the book, and their specific meanings in Britain.

NHS: National Health Service. In the United Kingdom, all healthcare is paid for by the government using public income-tax-derived monies. This means that all healthcare is free to patients at the point of delivery, whether they see a doctor in a local health centre, require an ambulance in an emergency, visit a hospital out-patient clinic, or are admitted to hospital for investigations and treatment.

Hospice: In 1967, Dame Cicely Saunders opened the first modern hospice, intended to deliver palliative care – care focused on quality of life at the end of life, rather than on extending life expectancy at the cost of any quality. She was building on the example of tender terminal care she had witnessed in St Joseph's Home for the Dying in Hackney, London, in the 1950s.

Hospices were a political reaction against the 'treatment whatever the burden' philosophy of cancer care in the 1960s. They were largely charitable institutions that worked in collaboration with local NHS partners, but rarely received NHS funding.

By the 1980s, UK hospices were specialising in whole-person care for people with incurable illnesses. Since then there has been a gradual shift from cancer-only services to care and expertise in reducing symptom burden for people with a wide variety of life-limiting conditions. NHS funding now partially supports the work of most hospices, and there is a national NHS strategy for palliative and end-of-life care that encourages cooperation between NHS and charitable providers of palliative care.

It is worth noting that, in the UK, hospices are mainly specialist units for management of complex physical, emotional, social or spiritual needs, and not merely end-of-life-care nursing homes.

Palliative Care Team: As recognition of the value of palliative care has grown, hospices have been unable to provide the advice and support needed across the country. Teams of palliative care specialist nurses, supported by a doctor with specialist training in palliative medicine, and often also by other experts in fields like physiotherapy, social work and chaplaincy, have been established both in hospitals, where they offer a consultation service to all wards and departments, and in the community, where they visit patients at home and advise their primary care team about symptom management.

Ward: Hospitals and hospices have in-patient areas, which may include single rooms or bays with several beds. The 'ward' is the whole collection of beds that is supervised and cared for by a single team of nurses. When I first qualified, we largely used 'Nightingale wards' in the NHS: long wards with two rows of beds, with the sickest patients closest to the nurses' station, from where all patients were visible to the nurse in charge. Modern hospital wards are divided into smaller bays, which provide more privacy for patients, but make it harder for the nursing team to maintain surveillance of the sickest.

Sister: The nurse in overall charge of a ward, a department or a community nursing team is the Sister (or charge nurse if male). The title is probably a remnant from the days of nursing orders of nuns. 'Sister' is in charge of the whole team, and responsible for the standards and outcomes of nursing care twenty-four hours a day. Although gradually being replaced by the term 'charge nurse', the title of 'Sister' is used with great respect (and usually affection) by public and staff alike.

GP (General Practitioner): A community-based doctor with expertise in managing the health of adults, children and babies. Usually working at a health centre (often referred to as a **surgery**) in teams supported by nurses and possibly also by pharmacists, physiotherapists and other expert clinicians. The GP is the first point of call for routine medical queries, and is responsible for a patient's ongoing care after discharge from hospital. They are trained to maintain a breadth of medical knowledge and skill in a wide variety of disciplines.

Primary Care: Care run and administered by health and social care professionals based in the patient's home, health centre or other community setting. **Secondary care** is hospital-based, and highly specialised treatments, only available in specific hospitals, are referred to as **tertiary care**.

Cognitive Behaviour Therapy (CBT): A psychological therapy approach initially developed to help those with emotional disorders like depression, anxiety, obsessive-compulsive disorder or panic, CBT helps people to identify how their thoughts and actions are triggering or maintaining their emotional distress, and to learn strategies that restore their emotional balance. Since the 1990s CBT has also been shown to be effective in helping people who are coping with physical illnesses, by building their resilience, their coping skills or their strategies for dealing with the effects of their condition.

DNACPR: 'Do not attempt Cardio-Pulmonary Resuscitation' is a medical order that is made when, for one or more of a variety of reasons, it has been decided that resuscitation efforts should not be made if a person's heart stops beating and/or they stop breathing. This allows natural dying to proceed. Reasons for a DNACPR order may include the patient's own preferences and decision, or a medical decision that their physical state is so frail that they would not respond to resuscitation attempts.

A DNACPR order does not refer to any other treatments apart from resuscitation: all other treatments should proceed as usual, for the benefit of the patient, unless they have been specifically declined by the patient, or have been deemed unnecessary by their medical advisers following a **Best Interests Decision**.

Best Interests Decision: Refers to making a decision on behalf of an adult who does not have the mental capacity to make that decision for him/herself. Under English law, the decision-maker must take into account any known views or wishes of the patient. These views and preferences may have been recorded by the patient in writing, or told to someone they trust, or may simply be reports of conversations with family and friends. The process is intended to try to reach the decision that the patient would have made, had s/he had the capacity to do so.

Resources and Helpful Information

Throughout this book, I have referred to a variety of places where the reader can find more information or read further around specific subjects. Here is a selection of helpful resources.

Dying Matters is a UK collaboration between multiple agencies and organisations that offer expertise in end-of-life care and bereavement. Its website offers easy-to-use materials about understanding and planning for the end of life. For example, for support and encouragement in discussion of death and dying, search for 'Resources – talking about dying'. For help with the making, storing and communicating of plans, search for 'Resources – making plans' and follow the links. See www.dyingmatters.org.

Mind is a mental health charity that offers useful resources for a variety of situations, including low mood, anxiety, panic, and flashbacks or post-traumatic stress disorder. Its website provides information about building resilience, and different coping styles. See http://www.mind.org.uk.

Death Café is a movement where an informal group of people gets together to discuss aspects of dying. Always welcoming, never judgemental, always with good cake. Its purpose is 'to increase awareness of death with a view to helping people make the most of their (finite) lives'. There are groups in more than forty countries. See http://deathcafe.com.

Planning in advance: Listen to Peter Saul, an Australian intensive care specialist, talking about this at https://www.ted.com/talks/peter_saul_lets_talk_about_dying.

Making a will is a good first step. In the UK, see www.gov.uk/make-will for advice. Many charities offer the help of a solicitor in exchange for a small legacy in the will.

Becoming a registered organ donor ensures that, if the circumstances allow, your still-healthy tissues or organs can be used to improve someone else's quality of life, or even save their life, after your death. More information at www.organdonation.nhs.uk.

There is information about making and storing plans for future care on the Dying Matters website.

Children's needs: For information about talking to children of different ages about dying and death, and supporting them in bereavement, there are helpful resources at www.dyingmatters.org; www.winstonswish.org.uk; and www.childbereavementuk.org.

Bereavement: Cruse offers listening support to the bereaved, and resources that include a website for young people and training for professionals who encounter the bereaved, including educators, health and care workers, and youth workers. See www.cruse.org.uk or www.crusescotland.org.uk.

Samaritans can be reached by telephone in the UK twenty-four hours a day. Trained volunteers will listen and help you to find help in your distress. www.samaritans.org.

For an insightful look at the process of working through bereavement, see Julia Samuel's beautifully readable book *Grief Works: Stories of Life, Death and Surviving* (Penguin, 2017).

Professionals: There is further information for health and care professionals from the UK's National Council for Palliative Care at www.ncpc.org.uk.

Perspectives beyond the obvious are discussed with skill by Averil Stedeford in her book *Facing Death: Patients, Families and Professionals* (Sobell Publications, 2nd edn 1994), based on her work as a liaison psychiatrist in a hospice.

People who are familiar with dying hear the same last messages repeatedly. Dr Ira Byok, an American palliative care physician and writer, has described how these core values of love, forgiveness, contrition and gratitude can support, repair and enhance human relationships in his book *The Four Things that Matter Most* (Simon & Schuster, 2014).

Atul Gwande's *Being Mortal* (Profile Books, 2014) is a moving account of a surgeon's insights into human ageing and mortality, and a clarion call for better discussions in public and professional worlds about mortality and the limits of medical intervention.

Letter Template

Wondering where to begin?

It can be difficult to open up a conversation about dying. It may be easier to start by talking about yourself, and your own wishes and preferences, before asking someone else what their ideas are. Making plans about future care may require the advice of a medical team, so the specific options can be explored. No such advice is needed, however, to explore those last messages of 'I love you,' 'I am sorry,' 'Thank you' and 'I forgive you.' You probably know already exactly to whom you would wish to say these things, but may wonder how to go about it. Perhaps writing to people may be easier than talking face to face, at least to open the conversation.

But how do you start such a letter? Telling people how important they are to us may feel daunting, as may asking for forgiveness or offering pardon for previous hurt. On pages 336-7 is a letter template. You could use this by photocopying the page and then writing on it, or you may prefer simply to use any ideas in it that are helpful to you, and write a letter in your own way to the people who are important to you. Then you might post it, or keep it and think a while, or read it aloud to the person. Or you could put it away for them to find and read after your death – but how much more benefit there could be for both of you to share it while you are still able to relish the new understanding such a letter may bring.

These resources are only that – resources. What you make of them, and of the rest of this book, is entirely up to you. I hope it helps.

Date ....

Dear ....

I want you to know that I have always appreciated

....
....

What I particularly love about you is

....
....

I hope you have forgiven me for

....
....

Please don't worry about

....
....

When you think about me, I hope you will remember

....

....

For your future, what I wish for you is

....

....

Thank you for being such an important part of my life.

Love from

....

My contact details:

....

....

Acknowledgements

There are many people to thank for their help and support in bringing this book into being.

First of all, I must thank every patient who has entrusted their care to the teams I have worked in. It has been my privilege to be their doctor for a part of their lives, and I am grateful for their trust. I have learned how to be a better doctor, and often a better person, from so many patient-teachers.

Thanks to the families who agreed to let me tell their stories. I have only been able to trace a few of you, but I was careful to do so when there seemed any likelihood that your story might be recognised. Your graciousness in dealing with my request, and your support for the project in granting permission, is very deeply appreciated.

I can't begin to thank the innumerable medical, nursing and other colleagues with whom I have had the pleasure of working over a career in medicine. Describing some of you in these pages, and reflecting on the fabulous contributions you make to patient care and to teamwork, has given me a warm glow while remembering our work together. I have changed all your names, but I suspect you will know who you are. Thank you for being my companions, teachers, allies and friends down the years.

A specific note of appreciation to the chairman and members of my local Clinical Ethics Advisory Group, for agreeing to devote a meeting to examining the issue of publishing patients' stories for public consumption, when patient permission was not possible. Although the General Medical Council guidance is clear about publishing clinical case reports to educate fellow professionals, the lines are less clear when the intended audience is not professional, yet the intention is public education rather than entertainment or gossip. Your thorough examination of the project, and your thoughtful comments, have made it easier to feel confident that this is a much-needed undertaking, and that with the safeguards I have been able to put in place, publication is ethically justifiable and morally acceptable.

The support of my agent, Andrew Gordon, was a vital contribution. Thanks for spotting the potential and then nurturing my efforts, and for your boundless enthusiasm for the project. I have David Schneider and Lucy Lunt at the BBC to thank for devising and skilful editing of a *One to One* interview on Radio 4 that piqued public interest and started the whole ball rolling. Little did we know what we were starting.

Friends and family have mulled ideas over with me, suggested books for me to read, commented on drafts, and made lots of cups of tea. Thanks, Josie Wright, for the use of your desk as a writing retreat, and for believing that I could turn the stories into a book. Tom and Jaclyn Bealer Wright, thank you for giving me time and space in your home in Quito so that I could spend quiet time writing, reflecting and watching hummingbirds.

The perceptive gifts of writing materials from Anne Pelham and Leonie Armstrong were put to good use in collecting my scattered thoughts and processing them into concrete ideas. And Anne Garland taught me how important a concrete idea is. Thanks, ladies.

I have had a wonderfully supportive reading group, whose comments, insights and suggestions have been essential: Alison Conner, Beda Higgins, Chris Wright, Christine Scott-Milton, Ellyn Peirson, Jaclyn Bealer Wright, Jane Peutrell, Josie Wright,

Lilias Alison, Lindsay Crack, Margie Jackson, Maureen Hitcham, Stephen Louw, Terri Lydiard and Tom Wright, thank you all for your thoughtful input.

The team at William Collins has been completely supportive to this project, from sympathetic design to enthusiastic promotion. Special thanks to Arabella Pike for gentle editing and firm encouragement, and Robert Lacey for detailed and sensitive line editing.

Most of all, I appreciate the quiet and unwavering support of my lifetime companion. Well-met on that corridor on our first day at medical school – I was lost with you on that day, and would have been lost without you ever since.

Kathryn Mannix
August 2017